FUNDAMENTALS OF SENSORINEURAL AUDITORY PATHOLOGY

Fundamentals of

Sensorineural

Auditory Pathology

By

WILLIAM B. DUBLIN, M.A., M.D.
Chief of Neuropathology and
Director, Laboratory of Auditory Pathology
Veterans Administration Hospital
Martinez, California
Associate Professor of Pathology
University of California
School of Medicine
Davis, California

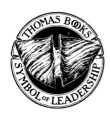

CHARLES C THOMAS · PUBLISHER
Springfield · Illinois · U.S.A.

Published and Distributed Throughout the World by
CHARLES C THOMAS • PUBLISHER
Bannerstone House
301-327 East Lawrence Avenue, Springfield, Illinois, U.S.A.

© *1976, by* CHARLES C THOMAS • PUBLISHER
ISBN 0-398-03507-5
Library of Congress Catalog Card Number: 75-26880

Printed in the United States of America
N-1

Library of Congress Cataloging in Publication Data

Dublin, William Brooks, 1909-
    Fundamentals of sensorineural auditory pathology.

    Bibliography: p.
    Includes index.
    1. Deafness.   2. Auditory pathways—Diseases.   3. Histology,
Pathological.   I. Title.   [DNLM: 1. Acoustic nerve—Pathology.
2. Auditory pathways—Pathology.   3. Labyrinth—Pathology. WV250
D814f]
RF293.D8   617.8'9   75-26880
ISBN 0-398-03507-5

to Our Family

PREFACE

T HIS WORK IS DEDICATED to the proposition that the central portion of the auditory pathway must be included in the meaningful histopathologic examination of cases of sensorineural hearing loss. In the past, while the inner ear has been studied extensive-
ly and an interest has been expressed in what might be found in
the brain, the latter purpose has not been brought to fulfillment.
As a result, the task has been only half completed. The project of
whole-auditory-pathway study has been impeded by lack of understanding of the cellular architecture of the auditory centers of the
brain so that a proper basis for evaluating the abnormal has not
been available. In recent years, however, advances in this regard
have been made in species other than man, furnishing the
stimulus and basis for similar studies in the human.

All too often, in the discussion that follows, the presentation
of pathologic information relative to the central nervous system is
unfruitful, but it appears that the time has come for an accounting
of normal structure, basic pathologic reactions, and those pathologic data that are available, in order to establish a base line
from which investigative efforts may be extended.

In the present work, descriptions are of human material, and
histologic sections are stained with hematoxylin and eosin, unless
specified otherwise. The terms in use in general pathology are employed, except where a structure or process is peculiar to the
auditory pathway. An attempt has been made to provide references to reasonably accessible publications in English. They are
not necessarily cited for documentation; indeed, the reference
quoted may in fact disagree with author's finding or interpretation. The latter is expressed without, necessarily, regard for
otologic tradition, but bearing in mind at all times the need for
bridging the hiatus between otologic pathology, neuropathology
and general pathology.

Considerable support has been given by various colleagues in the form of permission to reproduce certain classic illustrations, in some cases with the provision of original photographs. The publishers of concern have been similarly helpful. For this courtesy, the author is most grateful.

WBD

CONTENTS

FUNDAMENTALS OF SENSORINEURAL AUDITORY PATHOLOGY

Chapter 1 _____

METHODS

_____

General Principles of Organization—Public Relations

PREPARATORY PLANNING is indispensable to the proper execution of any histopathologic project. This is especially true of the study of the auditory pathway. There is great need not only for increased general interest in disease processes affecting hearing, but also for the establishment of lines of communication which will provide for the expeditious securing and processing of worthwhile material. The processing of auditory tissues is no small task if faithfully executed. Accordingly, the examination of a lesser number of appropriate cases will yield greater profit than the casual study of a larger amount of material, especially if the latter is inadequately prepared. Not only the diagnosis and treatment, but the histopathologic study of hearing disorders requires special interest and expertise. The services of special centers may be called on to advantage; however, the process of study must be carried out in such a way that the findings are properly correlated and are available to the various interested practitioners.

Various forms of expression of clinicopathologic interest are possible. The most important preparatory step doubtless is the establishment of audiometric records for correlation with pathologic findings. This forms the basis for a most valuable type of experiment.

One of the possible channels of procurement is to conduct the otologic study of patients who have difficulty in hearing and who suffer from presumably incurable malignant diseases. The bequest during life of temporal bones after death may be fruitful, providing that the bequest be made known to the physicians caring for the patients during their terminal illnesses so that on demise proper action can be instituted without delay.

3

If routine permission is granted for the performance of an autopsy without specified restriction, it is not legally required to secure special permission for the removal of temporal bones. The author contends, however, that not only do the surviving persons interested in the decedent deserve the satisfaction of knowing of the contribution made to medicine, but further, the overt recognition of the examination will tend to support general interest and confidence within the community. The examination of the brain is essential in every case of sensorineural hearing disorder. Prior discussion with responsible survivors and with the morticians, and the scope of the bequest, are framed accordingly with regard to the study of the auditory pathway and not just the removal of temporal bones.

Choice of Method in the Study of the Inner Ear

The different means of visualizing the structures of the peripheral hearing organ have their individual merits. For overall appraisal, especially when alteration in the bony capsule is anticipated, or when the status of structures other than those of the membranous labyrinth, such as the middle ear, must be accounted for, the step-sectioning of embedded tissue remains the procedure of choice. Whole tissue mounts in the form of surface preparations offer a decided advantage in the appraisal of the structures of the cochlear duct and their nerve and blood supply, and the methodology of the nineteenth century has been rediscovered (Johnsson and Hawkins, 1967). Transmission electron microscopy provides fine detail, although with restriction of size of field. Scanning electron microscopy adds the advantage of three-dimensional visualization (Bredberg, Ades and Engström, 1972; Lim and Lane, 1969). Undoubtedly, a combination of these techniques may be employed to advantage; indeed, some of the methods (see below) provide a degree of flexibility.

Removal of Auditory Tissues

The procedure for removal of temporal bones at autopsy has been outlined (Schuknecht, 1968a). Using the Stryker oscillating saw (blades of different sizes and shapes are available and may be found helpful), four cuts are made— (1) laterally, as close as possible to the temporal squame; (2) anteriorly, clearing the anterior surface of the petrous pyramid; (3) medially, clearing the auditory meatus; and (4) posteriorly, clearing the sigmoid sinus so as to include the endolymphatic sac (the dura should be left in place). The roughly rectangular bony fragment is delivered with chisel, knife or scissors, and forceps (the large Councilman bone-cutting forceps is helpful), keeping manipulation at a minimum in an effort to avoid fissuring and other such artifacts. If the remains are unembalmed, the cut ends of the internal carotid arteries should be dissected out and tied.

No special comment is required regarding removal of the brain aside from the obvious feature of gentle handling of the auditory nerve, which should be severed sharply to avoid avulsion from stretching.

Fixation

Optimal preparatory fixation of tissues is of the greatest importance. Owing to the notable tendency of the organ of Corti to undergo autolysis, fixation is of concern, especially in the study of the inner ear. Certain procedures and precautions have been suggested in combating autolysis. The remains should be refrigerated as soon as possible following demise, and autopsy should be conducted with a minimum of delay; a period of ten hours has been suggested as a time limit within which the organ of Corti will remain in usable condition (Bredberg, 1968). If a worker of suitable ability and responsibility is immediately available, 10 ml of 20 percent formalin can be injected slowly into the middle ear as soon as possible after death (Fernandez, 1958; Schuknecht, 1968a). Central nervous system tissues, while their condition naturally will be enhanced by prompt fixation, do not present so great a problem of autolysis as does the organ of Corti. Since fixation by injection is generally preferable to that by immersion, the embalming of the remains, done before autopsy and as soon as possible after demise, is a procedure of choice. This will expedite fixation of brain as well as of temporal bones. If possible, the autopsy should in such circumstances be delayed approximately four hours to permit action of the fixative. Prior embalming has the further advantage of making it unnecessary to secure the cut ends of the internal carotids and in most cases will be welcomed by the mortician, a colleague who can be an ally in this whole business if properly encouraged by considerate treatment.

The pertinent tissues should be fixed immediately upon removal. Refrigeration of temporal bones during the first day or two of fixation has been recommended. This implies that the action of autolytic agents will be retarded by lowering of temperature more than the rate of penetration of fixative will be. This principle could be reevaluated. Removal of the stapes has not expedited fixation as much as was hoped, and it may contribute to the production of artifact such as collapse of the wall of the membranous labyrinth (Fernandez, 1958). (Exception: procedure for surface preparations—see below.)

The choice of fixative varies with the technical method selected. For the standard step sectioning of embedded temporal bones, Heidenhain-Susa solution has been recommended (Schuknecht, 1968a). Its superiority over neutral (add a marble chip or fragment of blackboard chalk) 10 percent formalin could be subject to reevaluation; it is the author's feeling that in case of poor result, the differential between fixatives will not be chiefly to blame. The formalin solution is optimal for the brain.

Decalcification, Embedding and Sectioning of Temporal Bones

After fixation for a minimum of one week, temporal bones may be trimmed, if necessary, with a coping saw, and decalcification is begun in 1M EDTA (Birge and Imhoff, 1952) (Versene flake®—about 260 gm/L will suffice) brought to pH 7.40 with glacial acetic acid. About 250 ml of solution per temporal bone may be employed; it should be changed weekly. After one month, biweekly examination of the bones with X-ray (Hallpike and Cairns, 1938) is begun.* When no radiopacity remains, the speci-

*400 mas, 35 kvp, 36″ focus-film distance, cardboard holder and no filtration (Dublin, W.B., and Fraser, G.A.: *Medical Radiography and Photography, 47*:82, 1971).

men may be left in the EDTA solution an added two weeks to enhance removal of calcium that is too finely divided for visualization with X-ray. The margins of the bones may require final trimming; if gritting is still encountered, another two weeks of decalcification will be helpful.

The temporal bones are washed overnight in running water. Dehydration is carried out with daily steps of 50, 70, 80 (at this stage, the vertex of the bony pyramid is shaved horizontally so as to open the superior semicircular canal, to permit access of dehydrant, and later, of embedding medium, to the interior of the labyrinth), 90, 95 and 100 percent ethyl alcohol followed by a mixture of equal parts of absolute alcohol and ether. Infiltration with pyroxilin (Parlodion strips, Mallinckrodt) is carried out: 3 percent, ten days; 6 percent, fifteen days; 9 percent, twenty days; 12 percent, thirty days. Evaporation tends to lessen the jump in concentration of pyroxilin experienced at each step. Negative pressure expedites the infiltration (Donahue and Gussen, 1966); its use is thought to permit infiltration in much less than the time intervals just stated. The reduction of pressure can be achieved in the standard oven so equipped. A large glass dessicating jar with a well-fitting (ground) lid, using heavy stopcock grease, will serve if equipped with a manometer and a three-way stopcock. A non-explosive pump should be used or at least the outlet into the room atmosphere should be removed as far as possible from static-producing switches and the pump. A flask can be inserted in line as a trap for mercury and oil. In avoiding production of artifact it is important to reduce pressure gently, not more than 2 cm of mercury at a time, with a maximum of 25 cm. Vigorous bubbling is to be avoided.

During infiltration the lid of the jar containing the specimen is closed lightly to permit escape of solvent. When infiltration has been completed the jar is removed from the vacuum chamber and is exposed to room air with the lid in place but loose. From evaporation of solvent, the pyroxilin solution will gradually thicken until it has a firm rubbery consistency. About 2 cm of chloroform is layered over the pyroxilin, and the latter is permitted to harden for two days. The block is preserved in 70 percent alcohol with a change or two to remove the bulk of the retained chloroform. At time of sectioning, a medium of 80 percent alcohol is employed for slight relative hardness.

The tissue is sectioned on a sliding microtome at twenty to twenty-five microns, the sections being preserved in 70 percent alcohol between numbered papers. Ordinarily every tenth section is stained, the remainder being held in reserve. Notching of a corner of the block will facilitate orientation at mounting.

Surface Preparations—Combined Methods—Phase and Electron Microscopy

Surface preparations (Engström, Ades and Andersson, 1966; Johnsson and Hawkins, 1967; Bredberg, 1968) provide continuity of histologic pattern. They are employed when only the tissues of the cochlear membranous labyrinth are to be studied, waiving information on the status of the other tissues such as the middle ear and otic capsule. In surface preparations, ganglion cells cannot be seen clearly unless the modiolus is sectioned (Johnsson, 1974). With the temporal bone *in situ,* or after its removal, the stapes is removed and the round window is opened, and the cochlear labyrinth is irrigated with osmic acid fixative. The bony covering of the cochlear coils is removed, and the soft tissues are lifted out, mounted and studied with phase and/or Nomarski interference contrast microscopy. Phase contrast yields good resolving power and is ideal for surface layer study. Interference contrast offers greater clarity at multiple levels, allowing minimal contamination from levels other than the one examined. The combined use of the two optical systems is advantageous (Kuhn, Thalmann and Marowitz, 1971). Various staining procedures can be employed, including that of Maillet for nerve fibers (Engström, Ades and Andersson, 1966; Bredberg, 1968). Tissues can, alternately, be embedded in acrylate for light microscopy or in epoxy resin for electron microscopy. Modifications have been offered (Bohne, 1972; Kimura, Schuknecht and Sando, 1964; Spoendlin and Brun, 1973) wherein the cochlea is embedded in plastic or resin and is sectioned *in situ* in half-turn portions and examined with phase microscopy; selected portions can be employed for light and electron microscopy. A procedural system has been developed that visualizes all intracochlear structures. It employs a combination of vascular injection, *in situ* fixation by perfusion, and decalcification, yielding surface mounts as well as sections (Axelsson, Miller and Holmquist, 1974).

Scanning electron microscopy has been employed to great advantage. This instrumentation is especially valuable in the study of surface preparations (Bredberg, Ades and Engström, 1972).

Technical Handling of Brain Tissue

For the most part, the technical handling of brain tissue requires no special comment. Most blocks of such material can be processed with paraffin technique with considerable increase in convenience over that with pyroxilin. Thicker tissue fragments can be left longer in the paraffin bath, as overnight. If entire brain stems are to be processed, pyroxilin may be employed with some reduction of infiltration time from that for temporal bones, as the supporting medium will diffuse more rapidly through brain tissue than through bone. The selection of blocks for study will be accounted for by virtue of the discussions of anatomy that follow later.

Staining Procedures

The use of unstained material for phase and interference contrast microscopy has been mentioned. For the routine study of sectioned material, hematoxylin-eosin remains a standard. Handling of pyroxilin sections is facilitated with the use of a small box containing a light source and covered with a ground glass; the hematoxylin solution is prepared by adding concentrated working solution to distilled water to a point just allowing visibility through the solution. This dilute concentration of hematoxylin works well for pyroxilin sections. An ordinary applicator stick serves conveniently as a carrier.

Added methods found to be applicable to the auditory pathway are employed in most histology laboratories. They include cresyl violet (Vogt) or thionin, protargol (Bodian) and luxol fast blue (Klüver-Barrera). These methods are described in the A.F.I.P. staining manual (Armed Forces Institute of Pathology,

1968). Since this standard publication is so easily available, the procedures will not be repeated here. One of the virtues of protargol is its reliability. Some other silver staining methods such as the Nauta-Gygax method for degenerating axons may be helpful on occasion (Rasmussen, 1957). Golgi preparations also may be of value in visualizing the dendritic pattern of nerve cells even though only a small percentage of neurons is well-impregnated (Geniec and Morest, 1971; Smith and Haglan, 1973).

Graphic Cochlear Reconstruction

The state of the sensory and neural elements of the cochlea may be depicted graphically in straight columns (Engström, Ades and Andersson, 1966) or in the form of a spiral (cochleogram). The latter may be constructed on a basis of distance from the base of the cochlea (Guild, 1921; Schuknecht, 1953) or in terms of radial degrees of the turns (Bredberg, 1968).

Chapter 2

DEVELOPMENTAL FEATURES

THE COCHLEA

THE MEMBRANOUS LABYRINTH (Arey, 1965; Anson, Warpeha, Donaldson and Rensink, 1968; Bredberg, 1968; Illum, 1972; Shambaugh, 1967a) first appears in the third week of gestation as a plate-like thickening of ectoderm, the auditory placode, situated midway on each side of the hindbrain. By growth and invagination the auditory pit is formed. By a process of continuing growth and closure the otocyst is produced; it soon separates from the overlying ectoderm. As the otocyst enlarges, the endolymphatic duct appears, at first arising from point of contact of otocyst with ectoderm, later shifting to a dorsomedial position. The central portion of the otocyst constricts to divide into the future utricle and saccule. At the point of division a relatively narrow segment persists as the continuous utricular and saccular ducts; these form a mutual junction with the endolymphatic duct. The latter produces a terminal expansion, the endolymphatic sac. This latter structure continues to grow after birth and into early adulthood; as the posterior cranial fossa enlarges, the endolymphatic sac, lying within the dura, is drawn caudally down the posterior surface of the petrous bone to a position partly overlying the sigmoid sinus.

At six weeks of gestation the cochlear duct begins as an evagination of the saccular division of the otocyst. By eight weeks the duct has elongated and has begun to coil; by eleven weeks nearly all of the two and three-fourths turns has been formed; after this the spiral increases some in size, but not appreciably in tortuosity. Cellular maturation of the cochlear duct begins near the basal end and proceeds in both directions, preponderantly apicalward. At the beginning of the third month the cochlear duct is oval, later becoming triangular when the vestibular mem-

11

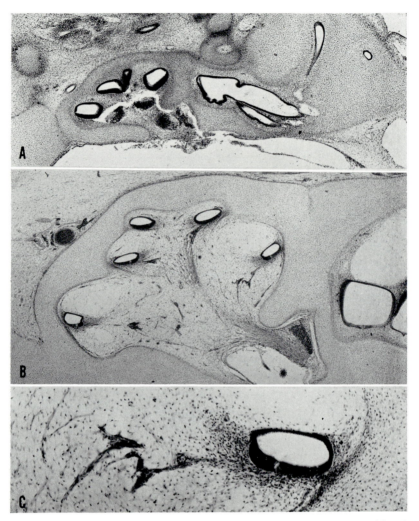

Figure 1A. Inner ear, embryo, about ten weeks of gestation. The cochlea is on the left with saccule next to the right, joined to the utricle. From the point of junction of the latter two, where there is a slight constriction, the endolymphatic duct extends, below; semicircular canals are to upper right. Spiral ganglion is seen in three cross-sectioned portions in region of future modiolus, centrally in the cochlea. Just to the right is a portion of vestibular ganglion. Cartilaginous anlage of otic capsule surrounds the soft tissue structures.

Figure 1B. Embryo, about twelve weeks. A somewhat similar view of cochlea and saccule with a portion of utricle. Immediately above saccule, perilymphatic space of vestibule is forming.

Figure 1C. Higher power view of a portion of cochlear duct and spiral ganglion from Figure 1B. Tunnel of Corti is beginning to form.

brane separates from the surrounding mesenchyme. At about twelve weeks the epithelium of the floor of the cochlear duct becomes thickened. Pseudostratification ensues, followed by differentiation into sensory and supporting cells. Inner hair cells differentiate before outer hair cells. Fluid spaces are formed. By about twenty-five weeks the organ of Corti resembles that of the adult. The fetus reacts to tonal stimulus with movement from the twenty-sixth week of pregnancy (Bredberg, 1968). The onset of

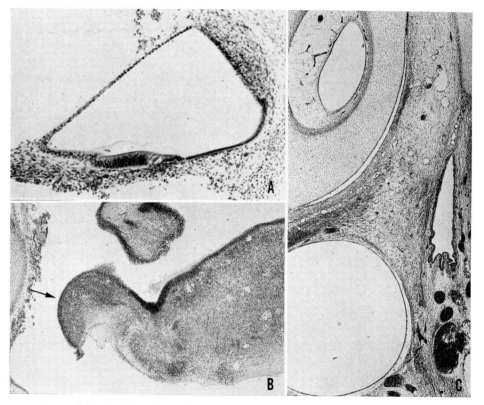

Figure 2A. Cochlear duct from embryo of fifteen weeks showing increased differentiation.

Figure 2B. Brain stem, eight-week embryo. Cochlear nucleus is developing on rim of alar plate (arrow).

Figure 2C. Endolymphatic duct and sac appear on right with some complexity of the sac (lower end of triangular space). Semicircular canal is at upper left, and sigmoid sinus, at lower left.

cochlear function is preceded by the opening of the tunnel space, formation of the spiral sulcus, differentiation and orientation of the tectorial membrane, myelination of nerve fibers and the formation of afferent and efferent neuroepithelial synapses (Pujol and Hilding, 1973).

The utricle and semicircular canals, the pars superior, well-developed at eight to nine weeks of gestation, are formed earlier than the saccule and cochlear duct, together constituting the pars inferior. Accordingly, the latter may be affected by pathogenic factors during gestation at a time when the pars superior is more fully differentiated and thus is less susceptible to injury. The pars inferior, further, has a later phylogenetic development. Following the general principle that phylogenetically younger systems are relatively vulnerable, the pars inferior may be comparatively prone to injury. This results in a concept of cochleosaccular degeneration (Paparella and Capps, 1973), the three main forms or sources of which are congenital or hereditary maldevelopment, viral infection and the aging process (Schuknecht, Igarashi and Gacek, 1965).

During its period of growth, the endolymphatic labyrinth becomes surrounded with mesenchyme. In the portion of the latter adjacent to the labyrinth, spaces appear which coalesce to form the perilymphatic space, containing supporting arachnoid-like tissue. Perilymph and endolymph come to fill the corresponding channels. In the cochlea, the perilymphatic space is represented by the scala vestibuli and scala tympani lying on either side of the cochlear duct. The perilymphatic connective tissue of this region is condensed to form the basilar membrane, separating the two scalae mentioned; in each of the latter channels, the perilymphatic tissue web is absent, permitting unimpeded vibratory movement of the fluid. The growth and differentiation of the perilymphatic membranous labyrinth are such that the mature proportions are achieved by midterm.

When the growth of the membranous labyrinth has been completed, the encasing capsule arises from the aforementioned enveloping mesenchyme, which becomes cartilaginous. On a plan not found elsewhere in the body, the cartilage is formed into three layers—an outer periosteal, middle endochondral and inner endosteal. These layers are transformed into bone. The periosteal layer thickens substantially following birth and continues into early adult life. The endosteal layer does not develop further; this would result in encroachment on the internal space of the cochlea.

In the endochondral layer, ossification begins about the margins of the cartilaginous lacunae. By birth this process has produced cancellous bone whose spicules appear in a background of embryonal cartilage (Fig. 3). Following birth, ossification continues until, by early adulthood, dense, poorly-vascularized, non-haversian bone containing residual cartilaginous lacunae has been formed. The cartilage islands remain identifiable throughout life. In this way the endochondral bone peculiarly embraces a retained primitive character while at the same time exhibiting petrous firmness.

The cochlear portion of the otic capsule develops in a spiral pattern parallel with the configuration of the organ of Corti. The central portion of the cochlea, the modiolus, similarly forms in a spiral reflecting the structure of the contained spiral ganglion and contemporary with the development of the cochlear duct. The modiolus develops directly from mesenchyme and is a membranous bone; it does not share the individualistic character of the otic capsule.

An ability to equalize pressure within the membranous labyrinth per se as well as in relation to that of the intracranial cavity is provided for by the formation of two bony channels through the wall of the otic capsule, the vestibular aqueduct giving passage to the previously mentioned endolymphatic duct, and the cochlear aqueduct (perilymphatic) containing arachnoidal connective tissue.

The internal auditory meatus and other such pertinent structures of the petrous bone are formed in relation to the development of the structures which they house or to which they give passage.

In the establishment of fetal circulation (Johnsson and Hawkins, 1972c) a dense temporary network of capillaries is formed. By selection and fusion the primitive plexus is transformed into larger vessels; unused parts atrophy. A large outer spiral vessel is provided; it is important for the development of the organ of Corti. It involutes toward the end of gestation parallel with the maturation of the hearing organ.

The bipolar neurons of the spiral ganglion and cochlear nerve (Arey, 1965) are derived from the primitive facial-acoustic ganglion. This cell cluster, situated just rostral to the otocyst, is of neural crest origin. A caudal portion of this cell mass, becoming the primitive acoustic ganglion, differentiates into superior and inferior portions. Some of the pars inferior takes part in the innervation of the utricle, saccule and semicircular ducts. The remainder differentiates into the spiral ganglion. This cell cluster rotates during its development to conform to the arrangement of the organ of Corti. The peripheral processes extend to supply the sensory cells; they are seen clearly even before the epithelium differentiates. Myelin is formed at about the 30 mm stage (Bredberg, 1968). The central processes form the cochlear division of the acoustic nerve.

THE CENTRAL NERVOUS SYSTEM

The cochlear nuclei (Arey, 1965) are gray cell masses of the central nervous system. Although situated superficially in the brain stem, they contain neurons of the second order and are not to be grouped with sensory ganglia. The wall of the primitive neural tube is divided by an internal midlateral groove, the sulcus limitans, into dorsal alar and ventral basal plates. The cochlear nuclear cluster is formed by focal proliferation of neuroblasts of the rhombic lip of the metencephalic alar plate. The cell aggregates thus formed are pushed ventrally. Certain other related cell clusters within the tegmentum of the brain stem also are derived from the alar plate.

The inferior colliculi originate from the alar plates of the mesencephalon. Proliferating neuroblasts migrate toward the surface of the colliculi and there organize into stratified ganglionic layers.

The medial geniculate bodies are of diencephalic origin,

again from alar plate tissues. The thalamus consists of a phylo-genetically older and smaller division, serving sensations of pleasure and pain, and a newer and much larger portion serving special and epicritic sensibilities. A particularly new portion is the metathalamus containing the geniculates.

The auditory cortex is formed by the proliferation of em-bryonic nerve cells of the phylogenetically newer part of the telencephalic wall, the neopallium.

Chapter 3 _____

ANATOMIC PRINCIPLES, WITH SOME FUNCTIONAL AND GENERAL PATHOLOGIC APPLICATIONS

O N THE AVERAGE, the auditory pathway is a connected series of about five neurons in addition to the sensory cells—those of the spiral ganglion, cochlear nucleus, dorsal olivary complex, inferior colliculus and medial geniculate body, the cortex serving as terminus.

THE COCHLEA

Gross

The petrous portion (pyramid) of the temporal bone (Bast and Anson, 1949; Bloom and Fawcett, 1968; Donaldson and Miller, 1973; Gray, 1966; Shambaugh, 1967a) is wedged in between the sphenoid and occipital bones. Its anterior surface forms the posterior part of the middle cranial fossa, and laterally it is continuous with the horizontal temporal squame. Its posterior surface forms the anterior part of the posterior cranial fossa. Near the medial border of the posterior surface the orifice of the internal acoustic meatus appears. The latter is about 1 cm in length. It transmits the acoustic and facial nerves, the nervus intermedius and the labyrinthine (internal auditory) artery. Lateral to the internal acoustic meatus is the orifice of the vestibular aqueduct (*see* Figure 3).

The petrous pyramid houses the inner ear, or labyrinth, consisting of two parts—osseous, a series of cavities, and membranous, a series of communicating sacs and ducts within the bony cavities

18

and containing the peripheral organs of hearing and equilibrium. In the adult the immediately investing osseous otic capsule is composed of bone of such hardness that the petrous bone surrounding it can be removed differentially as in an archeologic excavation.

The osseous labyrinth consists of three parts—the vestibule, semicircular canals and cochlea. The vestibule is the central part of the osseous labyrinth. It is somewhat ovoid in shape, flattened transversely. It contains the saccule and utricle. On its lateral wall, facing on the middle ear cavity, is the oval window, closed by the footplate of the stapes. Slightly posteroinferior to the oval window, placed at the bottom of a funnel-shaped depression, the round window niche, is the round window. It leads into the cochlea medially; it is closed by a membrane. Posteromedially the vestibule gives rise to the vestibular aqueduct. In the adult this structure is in the form of an inverted J with the curved end tilted anterolaterally (Ogura and Clemis, 1971). (The caudotropic force of growth of the otic capsule results in bending of the distal two thirds of the vestibular aqueduct at a point just behind the common crus.) It extends to the posterior surface of the pyramid. It gives passage to the endolymphatic duct, and terminally it expands to accommodate the first part of the endolymphatic sac. The perilymphatic space reaches the endolymphatic sac but does not extend into the posterior cranial fossa. A companion duct, the paravestibular canaliculus, is variably close to or distant from the aqueduct; it contains loose connective tissue supporting an artery and vein. Terminally, the vessels emerge from the canaliculus to supply the endolymphatic sac. The cochlear aqueduct arises from the scala tympani of the cochlear canal near its basal end and extends through the petrous bone to the inferior margin of its posterior surface in relation to the jugular bulb, establishing communication between the perilymphatic channel and the subarachnoid space.

The cochlea lies anteromedial to, and at its basal extremity communicates with, the vestibule. Its apex is directed forward, laterally and slightly downward. The cochlea is conical in form, measuring about 5 mm from base to apex and about 9 mm across at the base, and its canal is about 35 mm in length. As its name

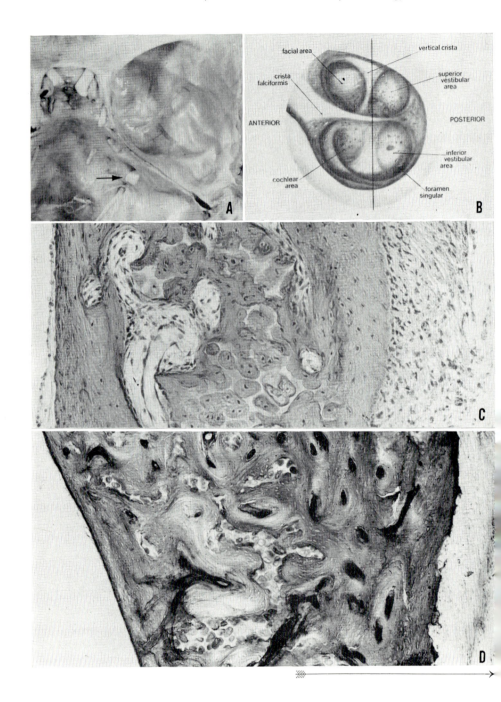

implies, the cochlea has a spiral structure, exhibiting two and three quarters turns. The spiral (viewed through the base) is clockwise on the right and counter clockwise on the left. At the base, the lower turn bends so as to present a concave centrifugal surface. The conical central axis of the cochlea is the modiolus, composed of comparatively spongy bone. Its base corresponds to the bottom of the internal auditory meatus which is closed by a bony plate, the lamina cribrosa. The latter is divided into two parts by a transverse ridge of bone, the crista falciformis. The anterior portion of the lower part is occupied by the aforementioned modiolar base, presenting a spiralling conical recess, and perforated by numerous orifices for passage of filaments of the cochlear nerve. The foramina successively bend outward, and by enlargement and confluence form the spiral canal of the modiolus (Rosenthal's canal) which lodges the spiral ganglion. From the margin of the modiolus there extends the osseous spiral lamina which partially divides the cochlear canal into two. The lamina consists of two thin plates of bone enclosing a central space in which nerve fibers and blood vessels course.

The cochlear canal is lined with endosteum; the latter serves as lining of the corresponding membranous ducts. Arachnoid-like membrane is not found in this canal, providing for unimpeded vibration of the contained fluid. The cochlear canal is divided by the joined osseous spiral lamina and basilar membrane into a superior scala vestibuli and an inferior scala tympani. These are perilymphatic ducts. The scala vestibuli joins the

Figure 3A. Portion of floor of skull showing inner ear with dural covering. Middle cranial fossa is above, and posterior fossa is below; sella is to upper left of the pyramid. Acoustic nerve (arrow) enters the internal acoustic meatus.

Figure 3B. Drawing of inner end of acoustic meatus. A spiralling, conical, perforated recess is seen (labelled *cochlear area*). After Amjad, Scheer and Rosenthal, *Arch Otolaryngol, 89:*709, 1969, copyright American Medical Association.

Figure 3C. Cross-section of wall of otic capsule of newborn. Endosteal layer is to left, periosteal is on right with endochondral in between, the latter showing cartilage cells.

Figure 3D. The same, adult. Cartilaginous remnants persist in endochondral layer.

perilymphatic space of the vestibule. The scala tympani ends at the round window. The two scalae communicate at the apex through the helicotrema. A third duct, the scala media (cochlear duct), is separated from the inferolateral portion of the scala vestibuli by the vestibular (Reissner's) membrane. This scala is endolymphatic. At its basal extremity it bends to terminate in a blind cecum; near the end of the scala media the latter communicates with the saccule through the ductus reuniens.

The endolymphatic duct arises from the junction of the utricular and saccular ducts; it extends through the vestibular aqueduct to the posterior aspect of the petrous pyramid where a terminal expansion of the duct, the endolymphatic sac, lies partly within the vestibular aqueduct and partly outside between layers of dura and overlying the sigmoid sinus.

Microscopic

The Osseous Otic Capsule

The bony otic capsule (Bloom and Fawcett, 1968; Donaldson and Miller, 1973; Gray, 1966; Shambaugh, 1967a) has an individually characteristic three-layered structure. The outer periosteal layer is composed of haversian bone as is the thin endosteal layer. The periosteum of the otic capsule is the dura. Endosteum serves as lining of the inner cavity of the cochlea. It tends to react to labyrinthitis or other source of tissue injury with the excessive production of bone that may occlude the inner ear completely (Altmann, 1965; Sugiura and Paparella, 1967). The middle endochondral layer is made up of bone in which cartilaginous lacunae remain from the embryonic stage throughout life. This bony layer is relatively inactive in reparative response; fractures involving the endochondral layer tend to heal slowly and sometimes never, showing only fibrous union.

The distribution of cartilaginous remnants characteristically includes the tissue adjoining a fissure which extends through the wall between the vestibule and the middle ear cavity just anterior to the oval window (fissula ante fenestram). This cleft contains an irregular ribbon of connective tissue. The fossula post fenestram, situated just behind the oval window, resembles the just-mentioned fissula but is smaller and less constant, being found in about two thirds of human ears, and as a complete fissure in 15 percent. It also is margined by embryonal cartilaginous rests.

The Membranous Labyrinth

The round window membrane is composed of an outer layer of flattened tympanic epithelium on a basal lamina and an intermediate collagenous and elastic connective tissue layer, the inner surface being covered by labyrinthine epithelial cells, representing the inner lining of the cochlea. The structure of the round window membrane does not indicate an active transport mechanism (Belluci, Fisher and Rhodin, 1972).

The cochlear aqueduct contains a sleeve of dura, and arachnoid-like tissue, including villi, representing an extension of the subarachnoid space. Avian erythrocytes injected experimentally into the subarachnoid space of the posterior fossa (cat) may be caught in the fine fibrous meshwork of the aqueduct; frequently some erythrocytes pass through into the perilymphatic space (scala tympani). The cochlear aqueduct is considered to be one of the provisions for equalizing pressure differences between the perilymphatic and subarachnoid spaces. Experimental occlusion of the aqueduct, however, was not followed by effects of consequence (Kimura, Schuknecht and Ota, 1974; Schuknecht and El Seifi, 1963; Suh and Cody, 1974).

As was indicated previously, the scalae vestibuli and tympani are freely open channels, devoid of trabecular arachnoid-like meshwork that could impede acoustic vibrations passing through the perilymph. The two scalae are lined by the endosteum of the otic capsule. They are separated by the spiral lamina. The latter is divided into an inner bony portion, the osseous spiral lamina, that extends from the modiolus, and an outer fibrous zone, the membranous spiral lamina or basilar membrane, that extends from the osseous spiral lamina to the lateral endocochlear wall, there attaching to the spiral crest (heretofore erroneously referred to as the spiral ligament; this structure does not possess the characteristics of a ligament, but is the product merely of differentiation of endosteum) (Bloom and Fawcett, 1968). The osseous spiral

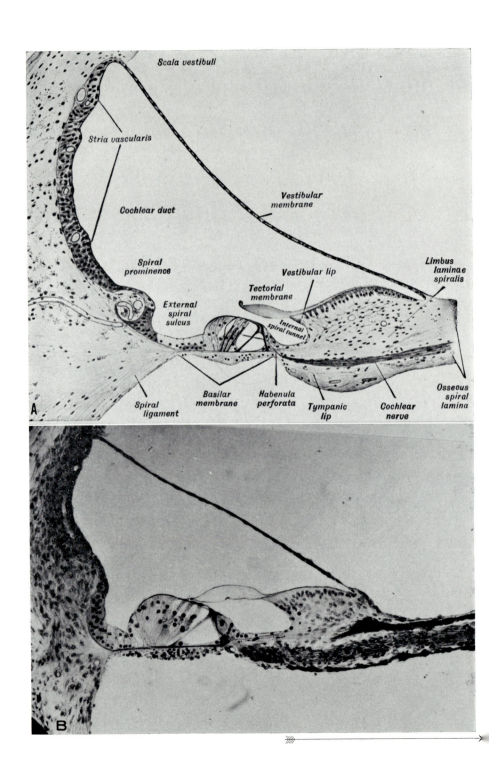

A

Scala vestibuli

Stria vascularis

Cochlear duct

Vestibular membrane

Spiral prominence

Vestibular lip

Limbus laminae spiralis

Tectorial membrane

External spiral sulcus

Internal spiral tunnel

Spiral ligament

Basilar membrane

Habenula perforata

Tympanic lip

Cochlear nerve

Osseous spiral lamina

B

lamina consists of thin upper and lower plates between which the vessels and nerves of supply course. The basilar membrane is composed of two sectors—a relatively thin central portion, the pars arcuata, extending approximately to a point beneath the outer pillar, and the remainder, thicker and striated, the pars pectinata. Some further details of fine structure have been observed with electron microscopy (Bloom and Fawcett, 1968). The basilar membrane increases in width from base to apex of the cochlea.

The cochlear duct (Bloom and Fawcett, 1968; Bredberg, 1968; Bredberg, Ades and Engström, 1972; Engström, Ades and Andersson, 1966), occupying the inferolateral portion of the scala vestibuli, is bounded by the vestibular membrane above and the wall of the cochlear canal laterally, and its floor consists of the basilar membrane and outer portion of the osseous spiral lamina.

The vestibular membrane extends from the osseous spiral lamina to the lateral wall of the cochlear canal. It consists of a basement membrane covered on each side by a cellular layer. The mesothelium on the upper side of the membrane is thin and flattened like that found generally in the perilymphatic system, and it is discontinuous. The epithelium covering the under surface of the membrane tends to be taller. In fetuses its pattern is even. In adulthood it becomes irregular with the formation of whorls and protrusions (Johnsson, 1971). On electron microscopy the epithelial cells present free surface microvilli (Bredberg, Ades and Engström, 1972) with pinocytotic vesicles, and basal infoldings are seen. Adenosine triphosphatase is demonstrable in the surface portion of the epithelium. The features are those characteristic of cells having a capacity for transport; the vestibular membrane can move sodium and potassium against gradients of increased concentration (Johnsson, 1971). Small inorganic molecules were found to pass through the membrane, while larger particles such

---

Figure 4A. Drawing of cochlear duct. After Bloom and Fawcett, *Textbook of Histology*, Ed. VIII, W. B. Saunders, 1962.
Figure 4B. Microphotograph of cochlear duct of squirrel monkey. Orient with 4A. Illustration courtesy Engström, Ades and Andersson, *Structural Pattern of the Organ of Corti*, Almqvist and Wiksells, 1966.

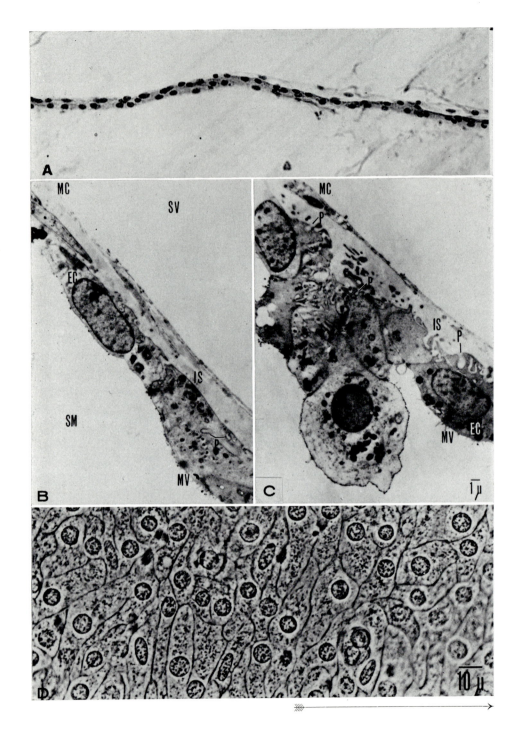

as albumin and colloidal gold did not (Mnich, 1971). Ferritin has been observed to pass from perilymph to endolymph, but not in the opposite direction, Hinojosa, 1971).

The stria vascularis covers the upper portion of the lateral wall of the cochlear duct. Its epithelium as seen with electron microscopy consists of dark and light cells (more, and less, electron dense). The dark cells exhibit deep basal infoldings; cytoplasmic organelles are abundant (Sugar, Engström and Stahle, 1972). Adenosine triphosphatase activity is found on the complex folds of the epithelial cells and on the surface facing the endolymph (Nakai and Hilding, 1966). These features are those expected in cells engaged in the active transport of ions and fluid. The injection of particulate matter has not resulted in pickup by the epithelium (Hinojosa and Rodriguez-Echandia, 1966). As its name implies, the stria is indeed vascular, and capillaries extend into the epithelial layer. The vascularity of the stria is comparatively simple or little developed in the apical coil; this increases to a status of rich vascular supply in the basal coil, suggesting a difference in metabolic activity along the cochlear duct (Perlman and Kimura, 1955; Sugar, Engström and Stahle, 1972). The foregoing features of the stria vascularis, as was indicated in relation to the epithelium, suggest a capacity for ion transport, and the organ is considered to be concerned with the production and the control, in a measure, of endolymph (*see* Figure 6).

In the connective tissue beneath the stria vascularis are cells

---

Figure 5A. Vestibular membrane. On the right, the upper, relatively thin mesothelial layer has been clarified by artifactious separation. Layer of cells lining under surface of membrane is thicker.

Figure 5B. Vestibular membrane, electron microphotograph. (MC) Mesothelial cells. (SV) Scala vestibuli. (SM) Scala media. (MV) Microvilli on surface of epithelial cells. (IS) Intercellular substance. (P) Pinocytotic vesicles. In Figure 5C an epithelilal cell is protruding into scala media. Numerous complicated infoldings and cytoplasmic processes are seen along basal side of epithelial cells.

Figure 5D. Electron microphotograph of surface preparation of vestibular membrane from five-year-old subject. A regular pattern is seen. Compare with Figure 73.

Figures 5B, C and D courtesy of Johnsson, *Ann Otol, 80*:425, 1971.

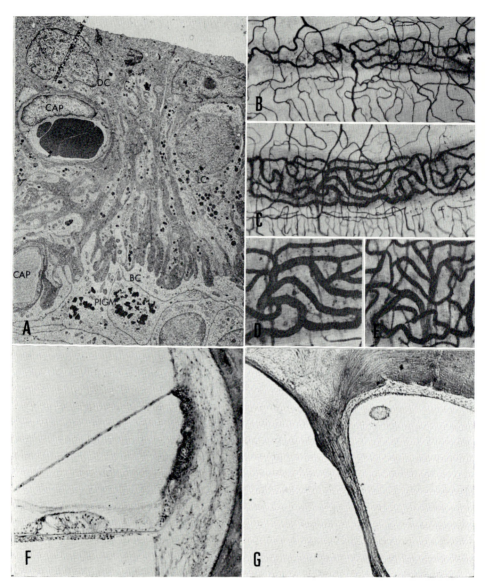

Figure 6A. Stria vascularis, electron microphotograph, squirrel monkey. (DC) Dark cell. (CAP) Capillary. (LC) Light cell. (BC) Basal cell. (PIGM) Pigment.

Figures 6B, C,D and E. Injection preparation of stria vascularis. A gradient

which can be seen with electron microscopy to contain granules that react with potassium dichromate at pH 4.1, indicating norepinephrine content. These cells are observed also in the connective tissue stroma of the spiral prominence. They tend to lie close to blood vessels. A role in vascular control has been suggested (Hilding, 1965).

The inferior portion of the stria vascularis is elevated somewhat owing to its extension down over the upper portion of the spiral prominence. This structure rests upon a richly vascularized thickening of the underlying periosteum. The epithelium covering the spiral prominence continues downward, dropping into a spiral sulcus, and continuing onto the upper surface of the basilar membrane. The cells here assume a cuboidal character, and those on the basilar membrane are known as the cells of Claudius. In parts of the basal coil, small groups of cells (of Boettcher) are interposed between the basilar membrane and the cells of Claudius.

The remainder of the space overlying the basilar membrane is occupied by the organ of Corti (Bloom and Fawcett, 1968; Bredberg, 1968; Donaldson and Miller, 1973; Engström, Ades and Bredberg, 1970; Engström, Ades and Andersson, 1966; Guild, 1937), composed of sensory and supporting cells together with adjacent epithelial cells.

The organ of Corti measures 33.5 mm in spiral length (Bredberg, 1968). It is divided into a smaller central and a larger peripheral part by the pillars that lean together at the top, forming the triangular inner tunnel of Corti. The fine structure of the pillars has been described in detail (Angelborg and Engström, 1972). On the central side is a single row of relatively short and flask-shaped inner hair cells, in total number ranging from 3,300 to 3,500. Each inner hair cell is supported and completely en-

---

of vascularity is seen from relatively avascular at apex (B) to more vascular at base (E). Figures 6A to E after Sugar, Engström and Stahle, *Acta Otolaryngol*, Suppl 301, 1972.

Figure 6F. Cochlear duct. (There is moderate autolysis of organ of Corti.) General features of stria vascularis are seen including large capillaries.

Figure 6G. Round window membrane, Bodian stain. A basement membrane is seen on each side with an intervening fibrillar layer.

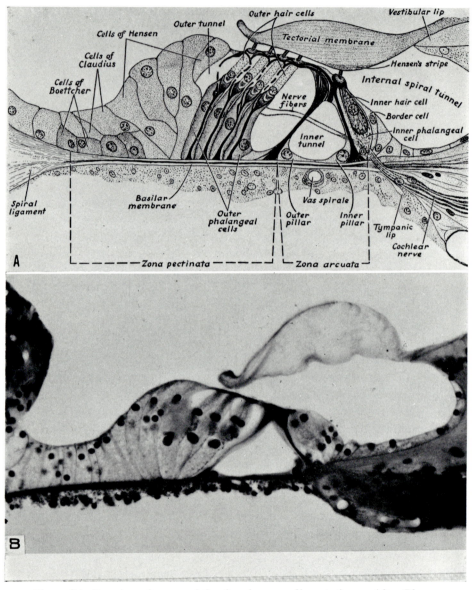

Figure 7A. Drawing of organ of Corti and some adjacent tissues. After Bloom and Fawcett, *Textbook of Histology,* Ed. IX. W. B. Saunders, 1968.

Figure 7B. Microphotograph of comparable structures, cat. Illustration courtesy Engström Ades and Andersson, *Structural Pattern of the Organ of Corti,* Almqvist and Wiksells, 1966.

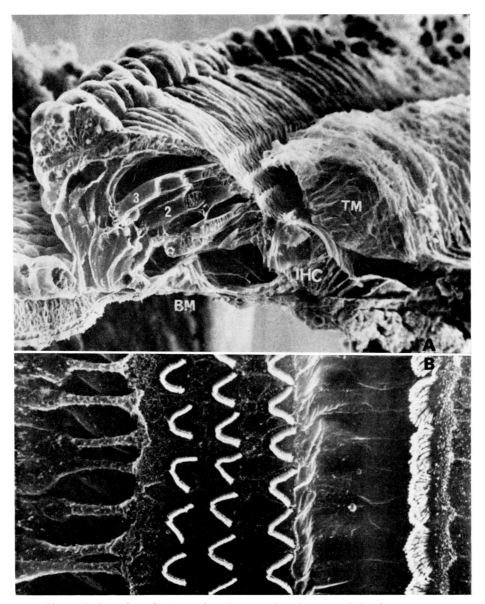

Figure 8. Scanning electron microphotographs of organ of Corti.
Figure 8A. (Guinea pig). (1,2,3) Rows of outer hair cells. (IHC) Inner hair
cells. (BM) Basilar membrane. (TM) Tectorial membrane.
Figure 8B. (Cat) Upper surface view. Phalangeal processes of third row of
Deiter's cells, on left (Hensen cells removed). Hairs of outer (3 rows) and
inner hair cells are seen.

Illustrations courtesy Bredberg, Ades and Engström, *Acta Otolaryngol,*
Suppl. 301, 1972.

veloped (except for the cuticular surface and points of application of nerve endings) by an inner phalangeal cell. Next to these cells in a central direction are border cells; they merge with the more flattened epithelium covering the inner spiral sulcus. The latter is a groove in the lateral border of the spiral limbus, a thickening of the periosteum covering the spiral osseous lamina, the groove being produced by the overhanging of the vestibular lip and the extension of the tympanic lip below. The latter extends just over the margin of the osseous spiral lamina and is perforated for the passage of nerve fibers.

On the outer side of the pillars are the cylindrically-shaped outer hair cells and their supporting elements, the outer phalangeal cells (Deiters). There are three rows of outer hair cells at the base of the cochlea, increasing to five at the apex. The outer hair cells range in number between 12,000 and 20,000. The phalangeal cells surround the basal third of the hair cells. They show a filamentous structure on scanning electron microscopy (Angelborg and Engström, 1972). The function of the phalangeal cells is more than merely supportive. They have been shown to be active in the pinocytotic transport of macromolecules and are well supplied with organelles; they appear to play an important role in the metabolic activity of the organ of Corti (de Lorenzo, Shirokyd and Cohn, 1973).

Lateral to the outer hair and supporting cells are the columnar Hensen's cells; they form the outer border of the organ of Corti.

Between the outer pillars and outer hair cells there is an open space of Nuel; between the outer hair cells and the cells of Hensen is the outer tunnel. The inner hair cells are contiguous with adjoining elements. The upper two thirds of the outer hair cells, however, are unattached and are exposed within a fluid-filled compartment that communicates with the two tunnels and the space of Nuel. The multilocular chamber thus formed is sealed off from the outside by the reticular membrane superiorly, Hensen's cells laterally, the basilar membrane inferiorly and the border cells medially. The fluid within the chamber is termed *cortilymph* (Engström, Ades and Andersson, 1966; Engström and Wersäll, 1953); it appears to have a certain individuality, al-

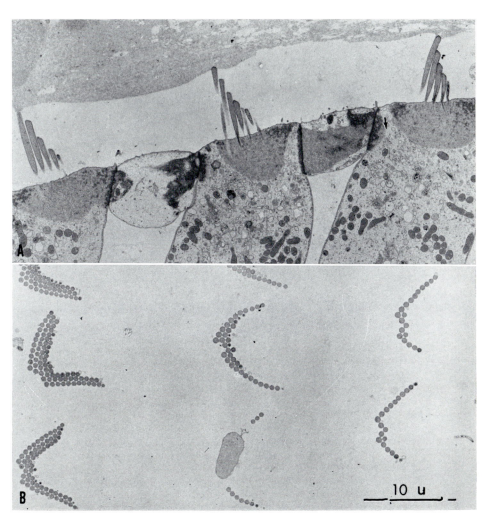

Figure 9. Electron microphotographs of hair cells showing the pattern of hairs.
Figure 9A. Section in long axis of hair cells (squirrel monkey).
Figure 9B. Hairs of outer hair cells seen from above (Rhesus monkey). See text.
Illustration, courtesy Kimura, *Acta Otolaryngol, 61:55,* 1966.

though communication with endolymph and perilymph appears to have a degree of freedom. The tectorial membrane is considered to be sealed to the Hensen cells and presents a barrier at an added level (Lawrence, 1974).

Passing toward the apex of the cochlea there is an increase in population density of hair cells per unit of spiral length of the cochlear duct, but a decrease in density per measured unit of width. The number of hair cells per unit of surface area is maximal at the base and decreases toward the apex. There is a nearly linear spatial distribution on the organ of Corti of the logarithmic frequency scale in the range from 500 to 32,000 cps (cat) (Schuknecht, 1960).

At their upper margins the hair cells are joined by the inner phalangeal cells and by processes extending upward from the lateral margins of the outer phalangeal cells in the production of a reticular membrane (probably contributed mainly by the phalangeal cells). Hairs (stereocilia) extend upward through the membrane (Kimura, 1966; Kimura, Schuknecht and Sando, 1964). They are arranged in the form of a W with the base of the W directed laterally, i.e. toward the Hensen cells. The tallest hairs are in the peripheral row of hairs (toward the Hensen cells), and the cells of the outer row of outer hair cells are taller. The taller hairs of outer hair cells are in contact with the under surface of the tectorial membrane. There is no firm evidence that hairs of inner hair cells are attached to the membrane; possibly they are not so directly involved in acoustic vibration.

The vibrations of the basilar membrane produce a shearing movement of the hairs of the sensory cells, thus initiating the process whereby the hair cells provide energy in the form of a stimulus to the nerve endings. It is considered that outer hair cells respond mainly to radial, and inner hair cells to longitudinal, shearing action (Spoendlin, 1967). Displacement of hairs during acoustic stimulation is considered to change the resistance of the cuticular plate, resulting in modulation of the electric current flowing through the hair cells (Honrubia, Strelioff and Ward, 1971). Ultrastructural techniques have been applied to the analysis of an electron transport system in hair cell mitochondria

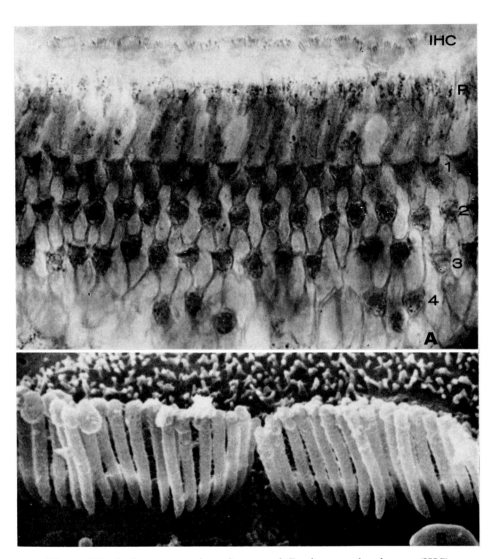

Figure 10A. Surface preparation of organ of Corti, upper basal turn. (IHC)
Row of Inner hair cells. (P) Phalanges. (1,2,3,4) Outer hair cells. Illustration
courtesy Bredberg, Ades and Engström, *Acta Otolaryngol,* Suppl. 236, 1968.
Figure 10B. Scanning electron microphotograph of hairs, cat. A few blebs
are seen on ends of normal hairs; they appear in greater numbers in noise
exposure. Illustration courtesy Bredberg, Ades and Engström, *Acta Otolaryngol,* Suppl. 301, 1972.

concerning oxido-reduction respiratory chain enzymes (Spector and Carr, 1974). Added details of fine structure of sensory cells are available in the references quoted. The dissection of single outer hair cells in the freeze-dried state with determination of weight and of some chemical constituents has been reported

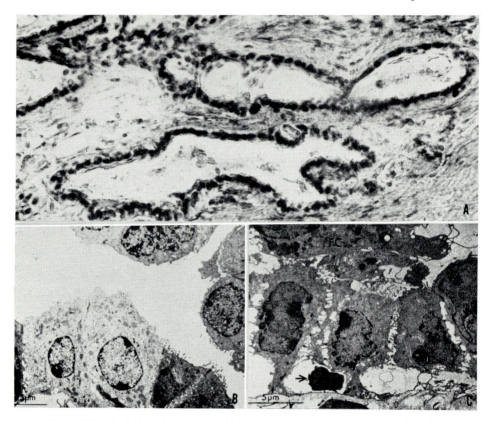

Figure 11A. Endolymphatic sac, middle portion, showing increase of surface area of epithelium by infolding. Underlying stroma is loose areolar and vascular.

Figure 11B. Electron microphotograph of sac epithelium from control animal (guinea pig) showing light and dark cells.

Figure 11C. Same, twenty-four hours after cryosurgery. The cells have become irregular with widened intercellular spaces and formation of filiform processes. A macrophage is seen interstitially (arrow). Free cells (FC) are present in the lumen. Figs. 11B, C after Schindler, Lundquist and Morrison, *Ann Otol, 83*:674, 1974.

(Thalmann, Thalmann and Comegys, 1972) .

The tectorial membrane is secreted from the luminal surfaces of the cells lining the upper margin of the spiral limbus. The membrane extends to lie over the organ of Corti, in contact with the hairs of the sensory cells as described previously. Fine structural details of the membrane have been reported (Lim, 1972) .

The endolymphatic duct (Lundquist, 1965) is lined by simple squamous or low cuboidal epithelium. The sac is divided into three sectors. In the proximal portion there is transition from the type of epithelium found in the duct to cells of more columnar type; however, there are no signs of special activity. The intermediate portion possesses tall cylindrical lining cells, and papillae and crypts are formed. The epithelial cells are of two types. Those appearing as light cells in electron microscopy are well equipped with cytoplasmic organelles. Pinocytotic vesicles and microvilli are seen. Basally, infoldings appear, presenting increased surface area. Dark cells have fewer organelles and pinocytotic vesicles, but appear able to perform phagocytosis. In the lumen of the sac, macrophages and debris are commonly found. The subepithelial areolar tissue exhibits rich capillary vascularity. The distal portion of the sac constitutes the third sector. Its lining gradually changes to low cuboidal; like the first portion of the sac, it does not appear to be functionally active.

The dynamic and chemical features of the labyrinthine fluids may be conveniently presented at this point. The fluids of the inner ear provide a medium for the metabolic exchange of nutriments and waste products within the organ of Corti, the maintenance of distribution of ions concerned with electric potentials, and the transmission of sound vibrations to the basilar membrane.

There has been considerable investigation, speculation and controversy regarding the relative participation of some of the previously described labyrinthine structures in the formation, maintenance (including pressure) , circulation and reabsorption of labyrinthine fluids and their chemical constituents. It appears that this activity is shared by the various aforementioned structures on a cooperative basis.

While perilymph requires homeostasis, it is not involved

strenuously in metabolic activity, and its relevant needs can be provided for by diffusion through the separating membranes.

The stria vascularis is thought to produce endolymph; comparison has been made with formation of cerebrospinal fluid. The stria vascularis is credited also with the passage of ions into the cochlear duct, hence the maintenance of electric potentials. Particulate matter introduced into the cochlear duct, however, has not been observed within the epithelium of the stria vascularis. Following the experimental rupture of the vestibular membrane by loud sounds, and employing a stain thought to be specific for endolymph, the mingling of perilymph with endolymph was found only in the region of the tear. With surgical incision of the vestibular membrane, little or no effect on the electrical response was observed basal to the tear. From this it has been concluded that the circulation of endolymph is local and radial (Lawrence, 1966a).

The epithelium on the under surface of the vestibular membrane is to be included with the stria vascularis in that it contributes in a degree to the dynamic and ionic regulation of endolymph.

The need of the organ of Corti for oxygen and nutriments is best served by the closest available blood supply—the capillary network beneath the basilar membrane, underlying the organ of Corti (Engström and Wersäll, 1953; Thalmann, Miyoshi and Thalmann, 1972). Degeneration of the organ of Corti follows destruction of the just-mentioned vessels but does not occur after injury to the stria vascularis (Lawrence, 1966c). The function of the phalangeal cells is more than merely supportive. These cells have shown pinocytotic activity and are richly supplied with organelles; they appear to play an important role in the metabolic activity of the organ of Corti (de Lorenzo, Shirokyd and Cohn, 1973). The cortilymph (Engström and Wersäll, 1953; Lawrence, 1969) has been so termed as distinct, notwithstanding the free diffusibility of certain substances, i.e. horseradish peroxidase, from the scala tympani (de Lorenzo, Shirokyd and Cohn, 1973) and cisterna magna (Duvall and Sutherland, 1972) through the basilar membrane. If an electrode is advanced upward through the basilar membrane and organ of Corti, the electrode shows a large negative potential at the level of the basilar membrane, zero at the level of the tectorial membrane, and then a sudden change to the large positive potential of the endolymph (Lawrence, 1969).

The endolymphatic duct and sac provide a means of removing fluid whose entry into the cochlear duct inevitably accompanies the transport of ions into the endolymph. The injection of iron ammonium citrate and potassium ferrocyanide into the membranous labyrinth was followed by the appearance of Prussian blue granules within the endolymphatic sac (Guild, 1927). Following the experimental introduction of colloidal suspension of silver into the scala media of the basal turn, silver appeared in significant amounts only in the endolymphatic sac, in macrophages and within lining epithelium. The light cells showed increased pinocytosis; the submucosal connective tissue became more cellular (Lundquist, 1965). Unlike other sacs of the membranous labyrinth, the endolymphatic sac characteristically contains debris. The participation of the endolymphatic duct and sac in a process of gradual fluid drainage and of the removal of particulate matter appears well-established. Obliteration of the duct and/or sac leads to endolymphatic hydrops (Guild, 1927; Kimura, 1967, 1968). The same effect results from blockage of the vestibular aqueduct (Kimura, Schuknecht and Ota, 1974; Suh and Cody, 1974). Following cryosurgical treatment of the lateral ampulla (guinea pig), signs of fluid reabsorption and phagocytosis of debris appeared in the endolymphatic sac (Schindler, Lundquist and Morrison, 1974). Filling and emptying of the intradural portion of the endolymphatic sac also provides a means of equilibration of cerebrospinal fluid and endolymphatic pressure (Arenberg, Marovitz and Shambaugh, 1970).

It seems reasonable to consider, in summary, that the stria vascularis governs the ionic, and to some extent the fluid, homeostasis of endolymph; the capillary network beneath the organ of Corti provides instantly-needed oxygen, enzymes and nutriments, and the endolymphatic sac participates in the absorption of fluid and effects the removal of particulate matter.

Endolymph has a high concentration of potassium ions, roughly thirty times that of perilymph; sodium, contrariwise, is about one-tenth that of perilymph (Smith, Lowry and Wu, 1954). The resting cochlear potential is considered to be related to concentration of the two ions and to the properties of the separating membranes. The resting potential of the organ of Corti is negative 80 mv; that of the endolymph is positive 80 mv (Lawrence, 1969). This stands in comparison with 2 or 3 mv in the perilymphatic fluid (Whitfield, 1967). If the cochlear duct is perfused with perilymph or with a solution with comparable content of potassium, the cochlear potential is depressed (Suga, Nakashima and Snow, 1970). The same happens following rupture of the vestibular membrane with admixture of perilymph with endolymph (Lawrence, 1969). Insulin hypoglycemia leads to decrease in endolymphatic potassium and rise in sodium; the high potassium-sodium ratio of endolymph appears to depend on an oxidative process ultimately utilizing glucose as source of energy (Mendelsohn and Roderique, 1972). Glucose levels are high in the organ of Corti. The processes of the inner ear on which ionic movement, electric potential and cell survival depend require oxidative metabolism with abundant resources of glycogen (Matschinsky and Thalmann, 1970; Spector and Lucente, 1974). Following acoustic stimulation, glycogen is depleted, especially in the outer hair cells (Stack and Webster, 1971).

The Cochlear Neurons

The nerve fibers found in the cochlea are of three types—afferent, efferent and sympathetic; the first two are myelinated. The afferent nerve fibers will be described in a centrifugal pattern, although functionally they are centripetal. The bipolar neurons of the spiral ganglion number about 30,000 (Rasmussen, 1940). Their dendrites or peripheral processes supply the hair cells of the organ of Corti; the axons or central processes form the cochlear nerve. The cell bodies are located within the spiral (Rosenthal's) canal of the modiolus. Their population density is greatest in the upper portion of the basal coil, decreasing toward base and apex (Bredberg, 1968). The modiolus is shorter than the cochlear duct. In most of the basal turn, nerve fibers run essentially

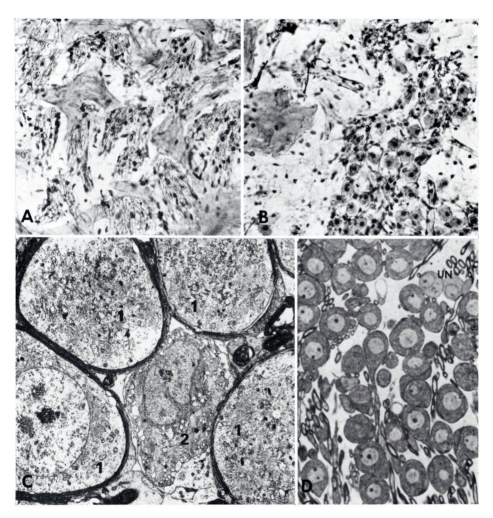

Figure 12. Spiral ganglion and intramodiolar neuronal processes.
Figure 12A. Axons within perforating channels.
Figure 12B. Cells of the spiral ganglion (newborn).
Figure 12C. Electron microphotograph of spiral ganglion, cat, showing the two types of cells (see text). Illustration courtesy Spoendlin, *Arch klin exp Ohr, - Nas - u Kehlk Heilk, 200:275,* 1971.
Figure 12D. Spiral ganglion of rat, toluidine blue, showing the main population of type I cells with two smaller, unmyelinated type II cells (UN). After Ross and Burkel, *Acta Otolaryngol, 76:*381, 1973.

straight radially, but approching the apex they fan upward increasingly; whereas frequencies below 500 cps are represented by the apical 20 percent of the organ of Corti, they are represented by neurons within the apical 10 percent of the spiral ganglion (cat) (Schuknecht, 1960). At the very end of the basal turn the nerve fibers slant slightly in a basal direction (Sando, 1965).

In certain animals, including the guinea pig (Kellerhals, Engström and Ades, 1967), rat (Rosenbluth, 1962) and cat (Spoendlin, 1971), the spiral ganglion cell bodies have been found to be of two types. Ninety to 95 percent (type I) are larger and are myelinated, and contain cytoplasmic vesicles. The remaining cells (type II) are smaller, possess thin myelin sheaths or none, and exhibit cytoplasmic neurofilaments. When the cochlear nerve is sectioned (cat) the type I cells and their processes degenerate, leaving the type II cells as survivors; the latter can then be seen more easily and clearly than in the normally populated spiral ganglion (Spoendlin, 1971). The dendrites of the type II cells are found to supply outer hair cells with the exception of a few (0.5% of the original cochlear dendrites) that take a radial course to the inner hair cells. The finding of the survival of nerve fibers under the foregoing circumstances obviates the apparent necessity for the previously-held untenable view that the peripheral fragments of processes that have lost connection with their parent cell bodies can survive by virtue of nourishment provided by supporting cells (Spoendlin, 1971). The nutritive capacity of the supporting cells, nevertheless, remains established and is demonstrated (in addition to previously presented features) by the survival of nerve fibers on occasion of the death of the hair cells supplied unless the supporting cells are also lost (Schuknecht, Benitez, Beekhuis, Igarashi and Singleton, 1962). Apart from the foregoing, a small percentage of spiral ganglion cells has been observed to be multipolar with ultrastructural features of, and found in the position of, parasympathetic nerve cells (Ross and Burkel, 1973).

The course and distribution of peripheral cochlear nerve fibers and endings is incompletely understood, remains subject to difference of opinion, and invites further investigation. The fibers are

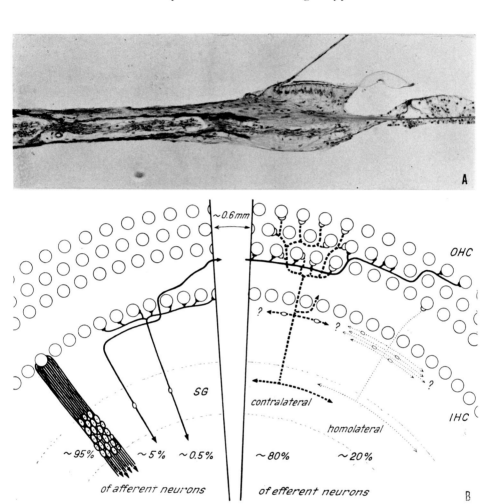

Figure 13A. Osseous spiral lamina on left with dendrites of spiral ganglion neurons between the two bony plates. The fibers emerge at the outer margin of the lamina to extend toward the organ of Corti.

Figure 13B. Diagram showing pattern of afferent fibers on left and efferent on right in relation to organ of Corti. The spiral fibers to outer hair cells extend across to the right. See text. Illustration courtesy Spoendlin, same source as in Figure 12.

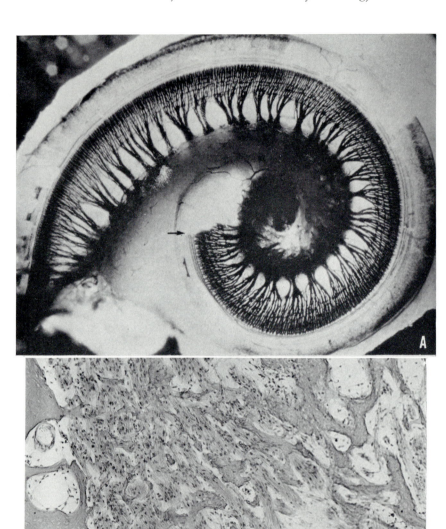

so closely arranged in the radial bundles that it is difficult to follow their course individually in whole-mount preparations, and
only limited segments can be followed in sections of embedded
tissues. Degeneration experiments like the one just described
(Spoendlin, 1971) are helpful, and pathologically comparable
human material would be valuable, especially if it did not involve
disruption of the cochlear nerve and if the brain stems were
available for study of surviving synaptic connections with the
cochlear nuclei. The following outline is offered tentatively.

The dendrites of the spiral ganglion neurons extend from the
modiolus, traveling within the osseous spiral lamina to emerge
through foramina at its lateral margin, at this point ceasing to be
myelinated; the fibers pass upward through the basilar membrane
and the peripheral margin of the tympanic lip of the spiral limbus, the latter extending just beyond the osseous spiral lamina
and perforated for the passage of the nerve fibers (habenula perforata) .

The fibers run certain basic courses, radial and spiral. Ninety
to 95 percent, originating from type I nerve cells, take a direct
radial course as the main supply to the inner hair cells (Engström
Ades and Bredberg, 1970; Lorente de No, 1937; Spoendlin, 1971).
These fibers are comparatively large in caliber. Each inner hair
cell receives terminals from twenty mainly unbranched nerve
fibers; each fiber supplies but one or two inner hair cells. A very
few radial fibers (about 0.5% of original spiral ganglion fibers),
arising from type II cells, pass to the bases of inner hair cells where
each fiber divides into two processes, the latter extending apicalward and basalward, respectively, to supply a total of some ten
inner hair cells. A few radial fibers pass to outer hair cells.

The spiral fibers comprise the remaining 5 to 10 percent of the
original total. Originating from type II nerve cells, they extend

---

Figure 14A. Whole-surface preparation of basal turn of cochlea, nerve stain.
There is normal, even distribution of nerve bundles. (There is reduction of
hair cells, apparently from cyclophosphamid toxicity.) Illustration courtesy
Bredberg, *Acta Otolaryngol,* Suppl. 236, 1968.
Figure 14B. Section through base of modiolus showing bundles of cochlear
nerve entering the tractus spiralis foraminosus.

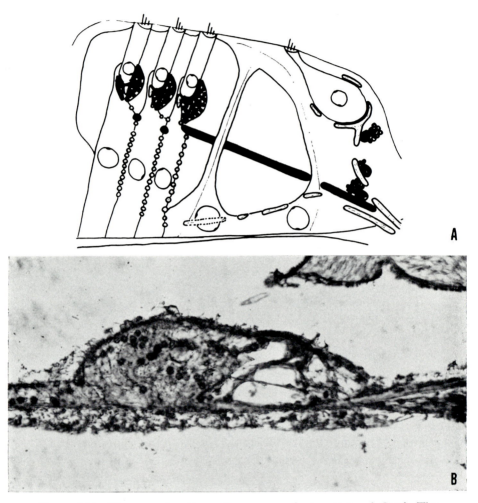

Figure 15A. Diagram of pattern of nerve supply to organ of Corti. The heavy line represents efferent fiber crossing tunnel to end in large, granular terminals. The other fibers are afferent (showing clear centers, lined on each side), supplying inner hair cell directly (radial), the dendrites to outer hair cells crossing at the bottom of the tunnel, and shown in cross section (circles) as spiral fibers coursing between supporting cells. After Spoendlin and Gacek, *Ann Otol*, 72:660, 1963.

Figure 15B. Organ of Corti, Bodian stain. Although especially the afferent fibers are seen but fragmentarily in a given plane, the general plan shown in the diagram is exhibited.

outward with the radial fibers, cross the bottom part of the tunnel of Corti, and turning basalward, extend as the outer spiral bundle for varying distances, as much as one-third of a turn, each fiber making contact along the way through collaterals with about ten outer hair cells. The fibers are wrapped (and appear to be functionally sustained) by the supporting cells (Deiters) and course between them along each row of outer hair cells (Spoendlin and Gacek, 1963). Alternate opinion indicates the upward spiral course of some fibers, the hair cells in general receiving their dominant afferent innervation from neural elements that lie radial to them; injury to the organ of Corti is followed by degeneration of radially-located spiral ganglion cells (cat) (Schuknecht, 1960).

The differences between types of nerve cells of the spiral ganglion and those between the patterns of nerve supply to inner and outer hair cells suggest the existence of two sensory systems (Kimura and Wersäll, 1962; Rosenbluth, 1962; Spoendlin, 1971, 1972). The inner hair cells could respond to a higher dynamic range while the outer hair cells could serve a function of spatial summation, providing greater sensitivity; however, especially sensitive fibers have not been found in the cochlear nerve (Kiang, 1965). A suggested alternate to the foregoing view is that the outer hair cells serve a function of control over the inner hair cells (Spoendlin, 1972). Loss of the service of the outer hair cell system could, accordingly, result in the development of loudness recruitment. The suggestion that outer hair cells serve a function other than that of primary auditory perception is borne out by the findings in acoustic trauma, where, with outer hair cells injured, the surviving inner hair cells have been found sufficient for maintenance of normal pure tone threshold (Ward and Duvall, 1971). The suggested functional multiplicity of hair cell systems, if it does exist, will support the concept of a capacity of the peripheral hearing organ for encoding.

Although with consideration of the foregoing, opinion exists that the innervation of, as well as the functions of, inner and outer hair cells presently remains debatable (Bredberg, 1968).

Efferent auditory fibers within the cochlea (Kimura and

Wersäll, 1962; Rasmussen, 1960; Spoendlin and Gacek, 1963)
represent the peripheral extension of the olivocochlear bundle,
and these efferent fibers and their branches and terminals degenerate if the bundle is sectioned. They course within the spiral
(Rosenthal's) canal as the intraganglionic spiral bundle, number-
ing some 500 fibers. These fibers extend outward with the radial
bundles. Some of the efferent fibers course beneath the inner hair
cells as the inner spiral bundle. Others cross the tunnel of Corti
at an upper level to supply outer hair cells. A spiral tunnel bundle runs beside the pillars within the tunnel; nerve fibers of the
tunnel type tend to be embedded in invaginations of supporting
cells (Spoendlin, 1969). The efferent fibers are arranged in a
fashion reciprocal to that of the afferents; they are predominantly
radial in relation to outer hair cells, but spiral in relation to inner
hair cells (Spoendlin, 1968). An enormous amount of branching
is required for the original 500 fibers to supply collaterals to the
many hair cells.

Encoding as a part of cochlear function is exemplified further
by the synapse of efferent fibers with afferents within the inner
spiral plexus, where a rich system of type II endings (see below) is
found. This permits regulatory or correlative action directly on
the afferent fibers in addition to the effect on the sensory cells
proper (Engström, Ades and Bredberg, 1970).

Nerve endings within the cochlear duct are attached to hair
cells on their modiolar side. The endings are of two types (Spoendlin, 1968) (not relative to types of spiral ganglion cell bodies)
—type I, afferent, relatively small and not heavily vesiculated, and
type II, efferent, relatively large and heavily vesiculated. The latter endings degenerate on sectioning the olivocochlear bundle.

The pattern of supply of hair cells with efferent endings is
variable. In the basal turn all three rows of outer hair cells exhibit endings; this gradually changes, passing toward the apex,
where the endings become smaller in, or disappear from, the outer row of outer hair cells and tend to be reduced in size in the
second row.

The efferent nerve fibers and endings exhibit acetylcholinesterase (Gacek, Nomura and Balogh, 1965; Iurato, Luciano, Pan-

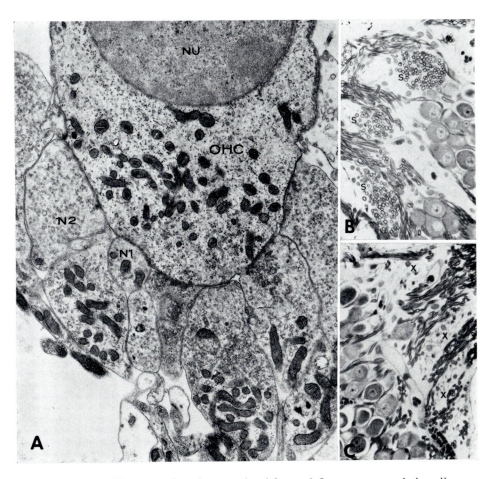

Figure 16A. Electron microphotograph of base of first row outer hair cell, guinea pig. (Ne1) Smaller afferent nerve ending. (Ne2) Larger granulated efferent ending. (Nu) Nucleus. (OHC) Outer hair cell. Illustration courtesy Bredberg, Ades and Engström, *Acta Otolaryngol*, Suppl. 301, 1972.

Figure 16B. Intraganglionic spiral bundle (cat) seen in cross section as small circles.

Figure 16C. Three weeks after sectioning of the olivocochlear bundle by transection of vestibular nerve. The efferent nature of the bundle is demonstrated by disappearance of fibers. After Spoendlin, *Acta Otolaryngol, 67:* 239, 1969.

nese and Reale, 1971; Shuknecht, Churchill and Doran, 1959). The reaction depends on the integrity of the olivocochlear bundle.

Adrenergic nerve fibers within the cochlea (Lawrence, 1969; Snow and Suga, 1973; Spoendlin, 1973) are thought to participate in the control of blood supply; they extend as far as the vas spirale. The source appears to be the superior cervical ganglion; histochemical fluorescence disappears following extirpation of the ganglion. Adrenergic fibers are also found apart from vessels, within the spiral ganglion (Ross 1971) and also in the habenular region where terminals have been found to make contact with afferent nerve fibers. Sound perception may be influenced through vasomotor control or by direct action on sensory neurons (Densert and Flock, 1974). Chromaffin granules containing norepinephrine have been found in cells beneath the epithelium of the stria vascularis; participation in the control of the vascular system is implicated (Hilding, 1965). Melanocytes are found throughout the labyrinth somewhat parallel with general pigmentation and tending to perivascular arrangement. A role in vascular control is postulated (La Ferriere, Arenberg, Hawkins and Johnsson, 1974). The demonstration of cholinergic nerve supply to blood vessels has proven elusive owing to difficulty of exclusion of other cholinergic fibers.

The cochlear nerve consists of the axons of the spiral ganglion. They pass centrally through the openings of the tractus spiralis foraminosus into the internal acoustic meatus where they are gathered together to form the cochlear nerve proper. The cochlear nerve is joined posteriorly by the vestibular nerve to form the acoustic nerve. The latter extends along the internal acoustic meatus and through the subarachnoid space to join the brain stem at the cerebellopontine recess formed by the junction of pons, medulla and cerebellum. At this point the cochlear nerve fibers pass over the dorsal, lateral and inferior margin of the restiform body and connect with the cochlear nucleus. In the internal acoustic meatus the nerve is surrounded by cerebrospinal fluid within pia-arachnoid in an extension of the subarachnoid space.

The cochlear nerve fibers initially take a spiral course around the cochlear axis, and this extends even into the free course of the nerve (Sando, 1965). Roughly speaking, fibers from the cochlear apex lie in the center of the nerve while those from the lower coils are more peripheral (Engström, Ades and Andersson, 1966; Sando, 1965). The tonotopic arrangement which this produces has been confirmed physiologically with the demonstration of progressive lowering of "best frequency" (frequency at which a given unit is activated at an intensity at which other frequencies are ineffective) as an electrode passes from the periphery to the center of the nerve (Kiang, Watanabe, Thomas and Clark, 1962). Unlike those of the cochlear nucleus, the electrical responses from units of the cochlear nerve are simple and uniform in pattern (Kiang, 1965).

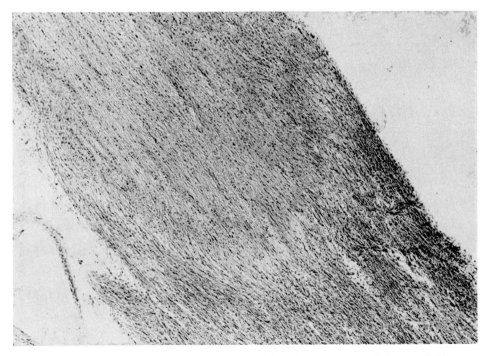

Figure 17. Cochlear nerve, showing transition between central (upper left) and peripheral (lower right) portions through the zone of the lamina c.i-brosa, the latter concave centrally.

The cochlear nerve presents a peripheral neurolemmal and a central glial part (Tarlov, 1937). The fibers of the former are supplied with Schwannian and endoneurial sheaths while the latter exhibit a "central" structure, being provided with glia, mainly oligodendrocytic. The central portion is likened to the optic nerve in being something of an extension of the white matter of the neuraxis (Hallpike, 1967). This portion of the nerve measures 10 to 13 mm in length in males and 7 to 10 mm in females. It undergoes transition to peripheral by passing through a lamina cribrosa (membrana perforata), usually but not always situated within the internal auditory meatus, and consisting of two sieve-like layers—glial and connective tissue—arranged in something of a shallow cone, concave centrally. The transition is not uniformly sharp and regular; fingers of glial-type nerve tissue may protrude on the distal side of the lamina. Less often, detached nests of glial cells may appear as much as 2 mm distal to the lamina. Myelin, as visualized on staining, is attenuated in the transition zone on the proximal side. Corpora amylacea tend characteristically to accumulate on the glial side of the lamina. The funicular pattern of the nerve as seen in cross-section varies among different individuals and among different regions of the same nerve. The number of fibers in the cochlear nerve ranges from about 23,000 to 40,000, averaging around 30,000 (Rasmussen, 1940). The number may differ between the two sides by as many as 5,000 fibers. The great majority of cochlear nerve fibers is myelinated, maintaining that character as far as the cochlear nucleus. A few unmyelinated fibers are closely associated with blood vessels and appear to be adrenergic, vasomotor. A few vestibular fibers tend to be included, especially marginally.

Blood Supply*

The labyrinthine (internal auditory) artery arises most often from the anterior inferior cerebellar, but it may take origin from the vertebral or basilar artery. It gives off branches to supply the acoustic nerve. On arriving in the internal acoustic meatus, the

*Axelsson, 1968; Lawrence, 1969; Smith, 1973.

labyrinthine artery divides to form the anterior vestibular and common cochlear. The latter in turn soon divides into the vesti-bulocochlear artery and the spiral modiolar artery (common coch-lear artery proper). The vestibulocochlear branch, on arriving in the basal turn of the modiolus, divides into vestibular and coch-lear branches. The former branch supplies the basal end of the cochlea and the vestibule. The cochlear branch supplies one quarter to one half of the basal turn and ends by anastomosing with the spiral modiolar artery. The latter runs upward in the spiral canal; it supplies nutrient branches to the spiral ganglion. Also, radiating arterioles extend outward at intervals. One group extends, in endosteum, over the scala vestibuli to the region of the lateral wall of the cochlear duct, there to supply the capillary systems of the stria vascularis and spiral prominence. The arteri-oles of the spiral crest are thin-walled compared with those of the modiolus, in whose walls muscle fibers appear (Kimura and Ota, 1974). The other group of arterioles extends through the osseous spiral lamina to the inner part of the basilar membrane; it sends branches to the spiral limbus and also forms the vas spirale be-neath the organ of Corti. Vessels are not found within the vesti-bular membrane, tectorial membrane or zona pectinata of the basilar membrane. Gradual reduction in diameter from small arteries to arterioles, and passage through long, narrow arterioles converts the pulsatile flow to continuous, possibly explaining why the flow of blood in the cochlea is not heard (Perlman and Kimura, 1955).

The role of the spiral vessels beneath the organ of Corti in supplying nutriment, whose immediate availability is essential, was presented previously. Experimental occlusion of the arteriole to the spiral crest and related structures (Lawrence, 1966c) re-sulted in degeneration of the stria vascularis and the cells within the spiral crest. The organ of Corti appeared to be uninjured. Occlusion of the branch to limbus and basilar membrane, on the other hand, resulted in degeneration of hair cells in the zone affected and of the limbus.

The course of venous return of blood flow (Axelsson, 1968) is difficult to outline with clarity owing to variation of opinion

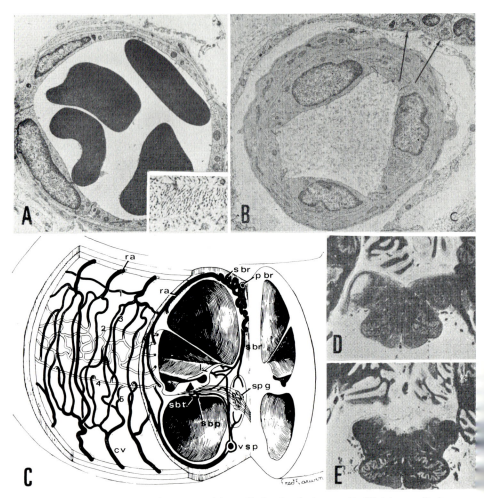

Figure 18 A & B. Arterioles. A. Thin walled, of spiral crest. B. Thicker-walled, of modiolus. Arrows indicate unmyelinated nerve fibers surrounded by Schwann cell. (C): Collagenous fibers. After Kimura, *Acta Otolaryngol, 77*:231, 1974. Figure 18C. Schematic drawing of blood supply to cochlea, guinea pig. (pbr) Primary branch of labyrinthine artery. (sbr) Secondary branch. (ra) Radiating arteriole. (1) Capillaries in upper spiral crest. (2) Network of the stria vascularis. (3) Arteriovenous arcades. (4) Capillary in spiral prominence. (5) Capillary in lower spiral crest. (cv) Collecting venule. (sbp) Spiral border beneath the tunnel. (vsp) Posterior spiral vein. (spg) Spiral ganglion. (spp)

and of resultant nomenclature and a tendency toward complexity and variability of arrangement of the vessels. Generally speaking, a double venous system consisting of anterior and posterior spiral veins coursing in the spiral canal receives tributaries from each of the three main regions of arteriolar supply—from the organ of Corti and spiral limbus through the osseous spiral lamina, from the stria vascularis and other structures of the lateral wall of the cochlear duct by way of the endosteum of the scala tympani, and from the spiral ganglion somewhat directly. The spiral veins unite to form a common modiolar vein; at the base of the modiolus the common modiolar vein unites with the vestibulocochlear vein and the vein of the round window to form the vein of the cochlear aqueduct. The latter drains into the jugular vein after passing through a pertinent portion of the petrous pyramid, receiving some tributaries on the way.

THE CENTRAL NERVOUS SYSTEM

The central portion of the auditory pathway consists of the cochlear and dorsal olivary nuclear complexes, inferior colliculi, medial geniculate bodies, auditory cortex and intercommunicating afferent and efferent nerve fiber tracts.

The Cochlear Nuclear Complex

Immediately central to the cochlear nucleus, crossing occurs of approximately half of the afferent nerve fibers; accordingly, this nuclear complex represents the centralmost neuronal structure whose injury may result in unilateral deafness.

The cochlear nucleus appears in man as a slight swelling of the cochlear nerve where the latter is attached to the dorsolateral surface of the brain stem at the junction of the pons with the

---

Spiral border below inner pillar. After Smith in de Lorenzo (Ed.): *Vascular Disorders and Hearing Defects,* University Park Press, 1973.
Figures 18 D & E. Occlusion of left posterior inferior cerebellar artery at two levels of medulla, myelin stain. The region of the cochlear nucleus with some adjacent structures is infarcted as shown by loss of dark staining reaction compared with opposite side. After Adams, *Arch Neurol Psychiatry,* 49:765, 1943, copyright American Medical Association.

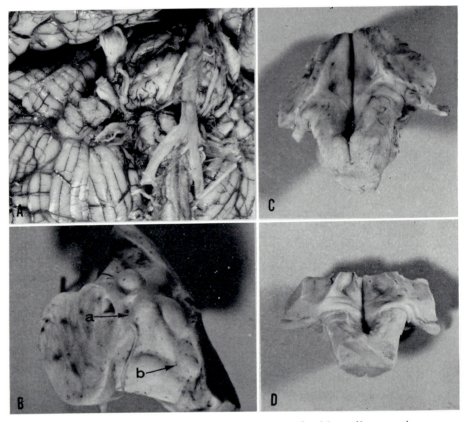

Figure 19. Gross features of brain stem concerned with auditory pathway.
Figure 19A. Cerebollopontine recess margined by cerebellum, pons and medulla.
Figure 19B. Pia-arachnoid has been removed from brain stem to show (a)
inferior colliculus, communicating through the brachium with (b) medial
geniculate body.
Figures 19 C & D. Dissection to show cochlear nerves and nuclei. In each
case, the usual adherence to the posteroinferior surface of the middle cerebellar peduncle is seen, especially on the left.

medulla. The nucleus is considerably attenuated in comparison
with its state in most lower animals. At its ventral extremity it
expands to about 2.5 mm, or perhaps slightly more, in cranio-
caudal width; it decreases to about 2 mm and becomes relatively

thin as it curves upward and medialward over the restiform body. The ventral portion of the nucleus is covered supralaterally by, and is variably adherent to, the middle cerebellar peduncle.

The cochlear nuclear complex is best visualized as a unit in sagittal section, although owing to its curvature, only the ventro-lateral portion of the dorsal subdivision is demonstrated in the same plane with the ventral nucleus.

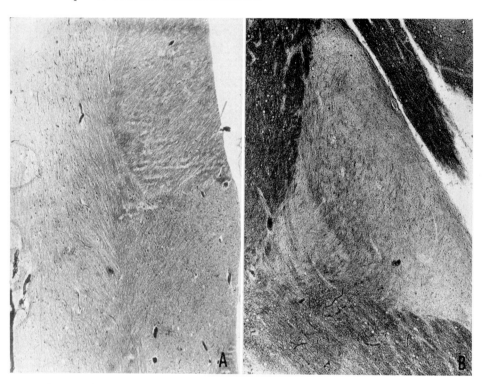

Figure 20A. Sagittal section of cochlear nucleus, Bodian stain, showing cochlear nerve fibers entering at midbottom, and dividing to send branches to superior ventral cochlear nucleus on right, and inferior ventral nucleus on left, some branches continuing upward toward dorsal nuclear subdivision, upper left, curving around restiform body, upper right. Compare with Figure 21.

Figure 20B. Transverse section of superior ventral cochlear nucleus, the latter appearing as large central, relatively pale triangular area. Weil myelin stain. Fibers are seen arching downward and medially to left; these fibers will participate in the formation of the trapezoid body.

Three subdivisions are recognized in the cochlear nuclear complex—dorsal, a somewhat attenuated ribbon, and superior and
inferior* ventral, the latter two being ovoid masses separated by
a hilum consisting of the root of the incoming cochlear nerve.
The cochlear nerve fibers divide into superior and inferior
branches. The former extend into the superior ventral nucleus;
the latter connect with the inferior ventral nucleus and send
collaterals to the dorsal nucleus (Lorente de No, 1933a).

Types of synaptic terminals of primary afferent cochlear nerve
fibers are important in relation to function. Single fibers carrying
single auditory impulses may deliver a complex of messages by the
termination of multiple branches in different types of endings on
different forms of neurons, each cell type receiving characteristic
types of terminals.

Calyceal synaptic terminals ("end-bulbs" of Held) imply an
express or through passage of the nerve impulse. This type of
nerve ending is large; it bears a resemblance to fingers grasping a
ball. The shrinkage attendant on processing could contribute to
the somewhat bar-like appearance of the processes. A single
calyceal terminal may cover much of the surface of a given cell
body; conversely, there is room for only a very few (if more than
one) calyceal terminals on a single perikaryon. Such cells are
supplied by a correspondingly limited number of cochlear nerve
fibers; provision is thus made for the firing of nerve cells by single
axonal processes (de Lorenzo, 1960a). Calyceal terminals make
firm synaptic contact at numerous points (de Lorenzo, 1960a;
Lenn and Reese, 1966). They make contact only with the peri-
karyons of neurons, not with their processes. This is understand-
able, considering relations of size and form. Less well-developed
types of calyceal synaptic terminals may be observed whose processes are variably thinner; such endings may approach more of
a basket form.

The other main type of synaptic terminal is a ring or bouton.
These round to ovoid, relatively small structures may appear,

---

*The terms *anterior* and *posterior,* employed in four-footed animals as synonymous
with cranial and caudal, become *superior* and *inferior* in man in consideration of
the erect anatomic position.

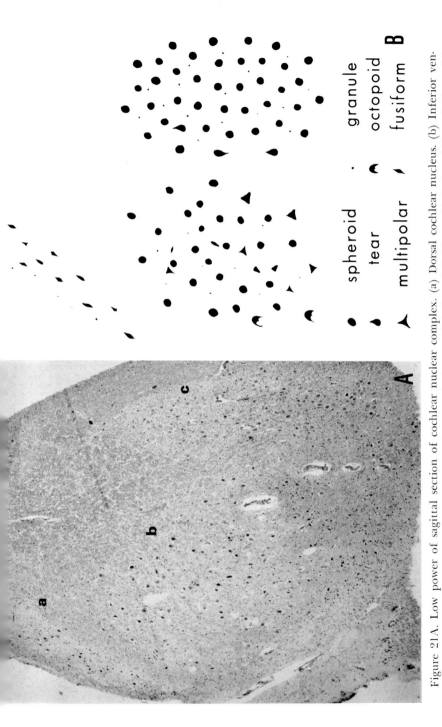

Figure 21A. Low power of sagittal section of cochlear nuclear complex. (a) Dorsal cochlear nucleus. (b) Inferior ventral. (c) Superior ventral. This illustration and those of Figures 23 A, B and C; Figure 24 A, B and D; and Figure 25 from Dublin, *Arch Otolaryngol, 100:*355, 1974, copyright American Medical Association. Figure 21B. Schematic diagram of distribution of the six nerve cell types found in the cochlear nuclear complex as encountered in Figure 21A. See text.

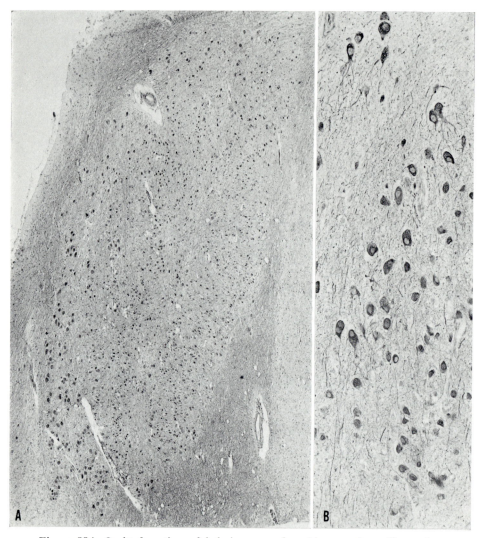

Figure 22A. Sagittal section of inferior ventral cochlear nucleus, illustrating variation in cellular architecture and exhibiting a marked degree of such variation. The nucleus is effectually subdivided into multiple cell clusters or portions. Along the inferior (left) margin where octopoid cells are customarily found is a field of large cells, subgiant in type, some of them multipolar and some suggestively octopoid. This abnormality had no apparent effect on hearing.

Figure 22B. The field at left margin is shown at higher magnification, Bodian stain.

sometimes in great numbers, on dendritic processes as well as cell bodies. They substantially account for the application of modifying impulses to nerve cells, although not necessarily being restricted to such a function. Efferent endings (as well as fibers) exhibit reaction to staining methods for acetylcholinesterase (Gacek, Nomura and Balogh, 1965; McDonald and Rasmussen, 1969, 1971, Osen and Roth, 1969; Rasmussen, 1964).

No primary cochlear afferents pass beyond the cochlear nuclei; however, many cells of the cochlear nuclear complex give rise to axons which run wholly within the nucleus (Whitfield, 1967). The incoming cochlear fibers supply all of the different nerve cell types. A reservation in this regard has been made in relation to the granular and molecular layers of the dorsal cochlear nucleus of the cat (Osen, 1969a), corresponding to the granule cells and the outward extending dendrites of the fusiform cells in the same nuclear division in the human (assuming that findings in the cat are applicable to man).

Different nerve cell types may be recognized in the cochlear nucleus of man. Considering that differences in neuronal structure should be reflected in functional differences, the nerve cell types stand suggestively as functional systems. Features other than those related to frequency alone must characterize these multiple systems. This view is in accord with the finding of variations among discharge patterns in different positions within the cochlear nucleus, supporting the concept of the cochlear nucleus as an encoding system, and not simply a relay station (Kiang, 1965). Further, there may be a correlation between regional distribution of types of neurons within the cochlear nucleus and discharge patterns in that, for example (cat), in the dorsolateral part of the anterior ventral subdivision of the nucleus (a location occupied preponderantly by large spherical cells as an essentially single-cell population), only one type of unit response was evoked, while in the central region of the ventral cochlear nucleus, where multiple cell types are intermingled, multiple types of discharge patterns were found (Kiang, Pfeiffer, Warr and Backus, 1965; Osen, 1969b). The location of the exploring electrode can, indeed, be determined on a basis of the just-mentioned correlation between distribution of types of neurons and discharge patterns (Moushegian, Rupert and Galambos, 1962).

The recognition of at least fifty nerve cell types in the cochlear nucleus has been suggested, although with limitation under conditions of practical application to two categories—large, with long axons, forming projection tracts, and small, having short axons, serving an intranuclear, integrative function (Lorente de No, 1933b). It seems preferable, at least pro tem, to establish a relatively simple system of classification on which to base further investigation into cellular architecture. This has been exemplified by the previous listing of nine neuronal categories in the cat (Osen, 1969a,b) and seven in man (Konigsmark, 1973).

Six nerve cell types may be recognized in the cochlear nuclear complex in the human, distributed in something of a regional pattern, although with considerable variation and overlapping of regions, and cells are frequently observed that are not clearly classifiable.

Spheroid cells are large, round to ovoid, and have abundant cytoplasm with prominent centrally or sometimes eccentrically placed nuclei. Rather delicate chromatophilic particles tend to appear in concentric perinuclear rings. In sections prepared with hematoxylin and eosin, dendrites are scant and twig-like. In Golgi preparations a spherical corona of numerous short dendritic processes appears; this structure is in contrast to the dendritic lamination of the inferior colliculus.

The spheroid cells are the chief populating constituents of the ventral cochlear nucleus. They are predominant especially in the superior ventral nucleus and appear also in the inferior ventral nuclear division, particularly in its dorsal portion, with variation. The spheroid (and other) cells are arranged more densely in the newborn than in the adult. This is owing to the amount of neuropil, which increases from birth to about age fifty and then declines (Konigsmark and Murphy, 1972).

The spheroid cells are supplied with well-developed calyceal terminals. These are seen best where cells are sectioned tangentially. Boutons appear in the spaces between calyceal processes; through them modifying impulses are received. Some of the bou-

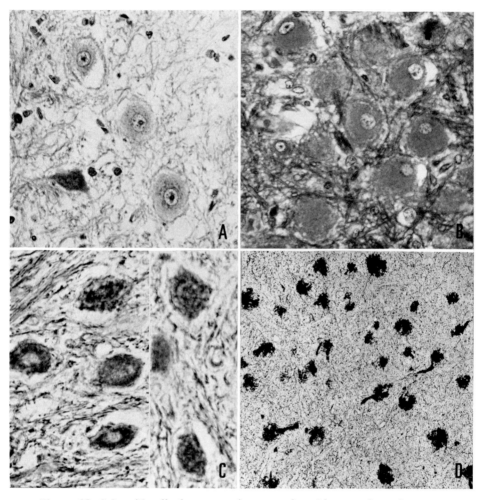

Figure 23. Spheroid cells from superior ventral cochlear nucleus. See text.

Figure 23A. Three such cells are shown with one incompletely demonstrated multipolar cell on lower left.

Figure 23B. Newborn. Toluidine blue. The intercellular tissue is comparatively small in bulk; it will increase with growth to adulthood.

Figure 23C. Two fields showing calcyceal synaptic terminals as network of irregular coarse bars. Boutons appear as small round to ovoid clear spots between the calcyceal processes. Bodian stain.

Figure 23D. Golgi preparation. The spheroid cells appear as rounded tufts; the dendrites are short and twig-like.

tons are acetylcholinesterase-positive (efferent) (Osen, 1970).

By virtue of numbers alone the spheroid cells appear to be the main second-order neurons of the afferent auditory pathway. The supply of but one or two synaptic terminals to each cell is in keeping with a capacity for fine frequency discrimination. The small spherical cells of the cochlear nucleus of the cat serve the wider range of frequencies of that species and are numerous in animals employing ultra high frequencies for echolocation, as the porpoise (Osen and Jansen, 1965) and bat (Hall, 1969). This cell type does not appear in the human distinctly and in numbers justifying recognition as a category. The reduced frequency range in man, served by the spheroid cells, is, however, attended by increase of integrative capacity. The functions of cells of large types other than spheroid are not well-understood, owing mainly to the rarity with which the individual cell types are injured selectively in pathologic states, and considering the difficulty attendant on the following of single secondary auditory fibers through the tracts to their destinations. It seems likely, but is unconfirmed, that the aforementioned integrative functions may be effected by the cells other than spheroid.

Tear cells are so named owing to their teardrop outline. They have about the same greatest dimension as spheroid cells, resembling the latter except for outline, and in some cases they are not clearly distinguishable from them. They receive calyceal terminals whose processes tend to be slightly finer than those of terminals on spheroid cells. (Reports vary as to endings found on tear cells in lower animals, ranging from "end-bulbs of Held" [rat and guinea pig] to boutons [cat] [Osen, 1970].) Tear cells are supplied also with boutons situated in between the calyceal processes.

With considerable variation the tear cells have a relatively limited and characteristic region of distribution, being found especially in the inferior margin of the superior ventral cochlear nucleus and in the superior border of the hilum in relation to incoming cochlear nerve fibers. Tear cells are thought to send axons to the contralateral trapezoid nucleus, a center of unknown function (Osen, 1970).

Multipolar cells may appear anywhere in the cochlear nucleus

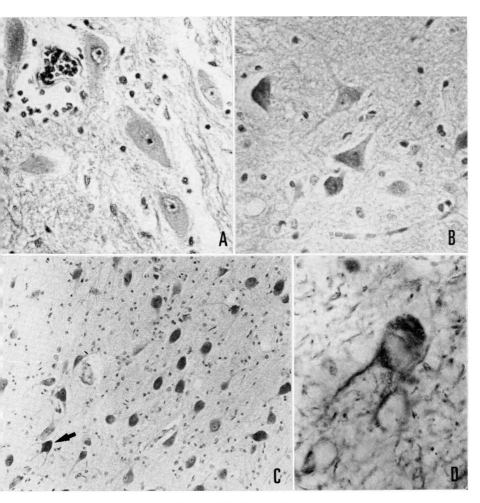

Figure 24A. Tear cells.

Figure 24B. Multipolar cells.

Figure 24C. Inferior ventral cochlear nucleus, cresyl violet, at the inferior and ventral margin. Octopoid cell indicated by arrow.

Figure 24D. Octopoid cell, Bodian stain. Boutons appear as small, essentially rounded, comparatively pale spots, most numerous over the middle one of three dendrites (the lower one is out of focus); a few appear on the cell body. Limited numbers of such structures are visualized in a given plane.

but are found especially in the inferior ventral subdivision, particularly in the ventral portion of the latter. Multipolar cells vary considerably in structure and could represent a heterogeneous complex. These cells in general are fairly large; they present the implied multipointed outline. Cytoplasm tends to be homogeneous and darkly staining, and a pyknotic appearance is seen, often without necessarily a pathologic implication. Multipolar cells receive calyceal terminals, suggestively still finer in texture than in the foregoing cell types. Boutons also are received in plentiful numbers. The multipolar cells project in the trapezoid body; their field of termination has not been established (Osen, 1970).

Octopoid cells (Osen, 1969b) are relatively few; they are found in the caudal pole of the inferior ventral cochlear nucleus. In sections prepared with hematoxylin and eosin or Nissl stains only scant portions of dendrites are seen. In protargol preparations the dendrites appear multiple, long and heavy, and tend to arise from one side of an individual cell body, presenting a drooping tentacular appearance leading to the designated term. As one would expect, calyceal terminals are not found; rather, only boutons appear in great numbers, covering dendrites as well as cell bodies. The features of small numbers of cells, multiple long dendrites, and supply of many synaptic terminals to individual cells suggest a broad-spectrum or, possibly, reflex function of the octopoid cells. The octopoid cell region in the cat has been found to send second-order fibers via the intermediate acoustic stria to certain nerve cell clusters in the periolivary region, considered to be point of origin of the olivocochlear bundle; the octopoid cells may conceivably represent the first unit of a feedback inhibitory mechanism (Osen, 1969a). Their injury could serve as basis for central recruitment (Hall in discussion of Dix and Hood, 1973).

Granule cells are the small neurons of the cochlear nucleus. They vary in size through a substantial range and doubtless constitute a heterogeneous group embracing a number of functional systems; points of division, however, cannot be made reasonably, and the inclusive categorical class is recognized at least tentatively. Granule cells are distributed widely throughout the

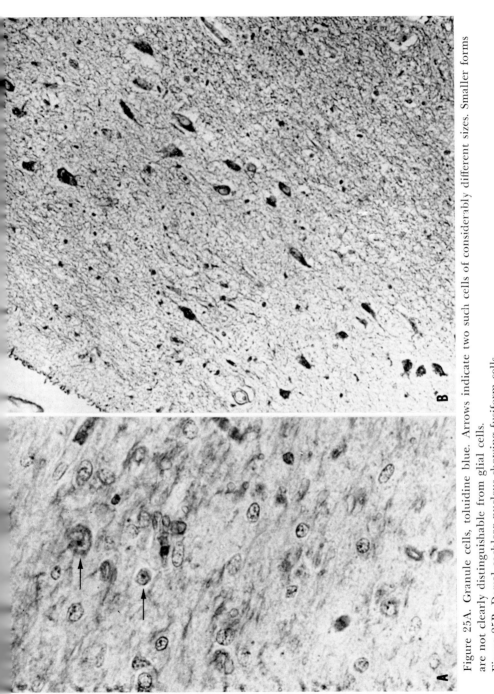

Figure 25A. Granule cells, toluidine blue. Arrows indicate two such cells of considerably different sizes. Smaller forms are not clearly distinguishable from glial cells.

Figure 25B. Dorsal cochlear nucleus showing fusiform cells.

cochlear nucleus. In the human they do not form as substantial a marginal mantle as in lower animals (Osen, 1969b). This is inclusively true of the dorsal cochlear nucleus, although in Golgi preparations a thin marginal layer is demonstrated. The granule cells appear to be Golgi type II, having short axons, and are thought to serve an intranuclear integrative function, perhaps effecting some connection between the nuclear subdivisions (Lorente de No, 1933b). In protargol preparations these cells appear to be supplied with basket-type terminals whose processes are simple and appear as thin rods or wires.

Fusiform cells may appear throughout the cochlear nuclear complex, but are found especially in the attenuated strip of cells representing the dorsal cochlear nucleus. Cell form in this nuclear subdivision may vary, including, in addition to fusiform, ovoid, tear or pyramidal types; fusiform expresses an average. Cytoplasm is stained evenly and deeply with hematoxylin and eosin. The cells tend generally to be oriented lengthwise along the longitudinal plane of the dorsal cochlear nucleus; there is some variation in this, and a few of the cells lie transversely, sending processes to the overlying granule cells. The well-developed laminar pattern observed in the cat (Osen, 1969a), however, is not observed appreciably in man in whom the dorsal cochlear nucleus appears rudimentary. The synaptic endings received by the fusiform cells are boutons. It is possible that these are from adjacent granule cells, the fusiform cells not being supplied with primary afferents (cat) (Osen, 1970). The fusiform cells are considered to project on the nuclei of the lateral lemniscus and the nucleus of the contralateral inferior colliculus via the dorsal acoustic stria (Osen, 1970; Strominger, 1969); this feature of apparent exclusive contralaterality is individually peculiar. The dorsal cochlear nucleus appears to comprise a somewhat primitive system, possibly reflex in nature. This would be in keeping also with the previously stated supply of fusiform cells with boutons.

Giant cells, found previously in the cat (Osen, 1969b) and in man (Konigsmark, 1973), are scarcely to be seen in the cochlear nucleus of the human and are not considered deserving of recognition as a cell type. These cells were not observed in the squirrel monkey or in six other primate species (Webster, 1971).

The Dorsal Olivary Nuclear Complex

Afferent nerve fibers leaving the cochlear nucleus all synapse at least once in cell groups somewhere between the pontomedullary junction and the midbrain (Stotler, 1953). (Possibly excepted are some fibers from the dorsal cochlear nucleus.) This group of nerve cell aggregates is referred to as the dorsal* olivary nuclear complex. This nuclear system represents the first station at which binaural integration in sound location is anatomically possible consequent to crossing of a roughly equal proportion of afferent auditory nerve fibers. Conversely, the chance of occurrence of unilateral deafness consequent to injury of the neurons of the region no longer exists.

Included in the dorsal olivary nuclear complex are the medial and lateral dorsal olivary nuclei, periolivary cells, trapezoid nuclei and nuclei of the lateral lemniscus. Some of these components are fairly well-defined and constant, others less so. The categorization of different large cell types within the individual centers of the complex is not practical.

In certain lower animals having a capacity for receiving a higher range of frequencies, i.e. cat, the principal superior olivary nucleus is the lateral subdivision (supplied by the small spherical cells of the ventral cochlear nucleus), seen as an S-shaped structure. A medially-situated accessory nucleus is small and functionally secondary. This state is emphasized in the bat (Hall, 1969) and porpoise (Osen and Jansen, 1965), wherein very high frequencies are employed for echolocation. The situation is reversed in primates, including especially man, in whom the frequency scale is reduced; the lateral dorsal olive regresses into an ill-defined, poorly-cellular group, and the accessory nucleus becomes predominant and is recognized as the medial dorsal olivary nucleus (Irving and Harrison, 1967; Stotler, 1953). This is accompanied by implementation of integration with other functional systems such as visual. The medial dorsal olivary nucleus is small or absent in animals with small eyes, but large in association with

---

*The terms *superior* and *inferior,* that in the horizontal position of four-footed animals are synonymous with the back and front, become *dorsal* and *ventral* in man whose anatomic position is vertical.

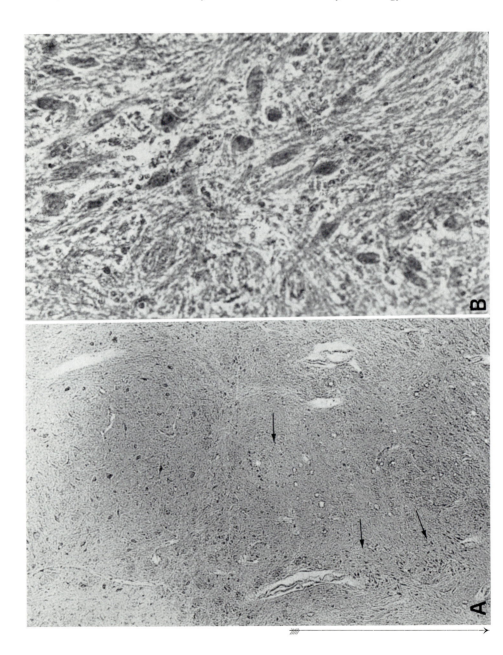

cone retinas, predominantly cone foveas, or rod retinas in large eyes (Irving and Harrison, 1967).

The medial dorsal olivary nucleus (supplied by the spheroid cells of the ventral cochlear nucleus) is in the form of an essentially rectangular, thin plate extending from the superior margin of the ventral olivary nucleus and inferior border of the facial nucleus, craniad for 4 mm, or slightly more, just beyond the superior margin of the facial nucleus. It lies just medial and ventral to the facial nucleus. As seen in transverse sections, the dorsal portion of the medial dorsal olivary nucleus lies in a vertical plane, the ventral portion bending laterally in a slight angle at about the midpoint. The nucleus is composed of a slightly stratified column of elongated fusiform neurons tending to be oriented lengthwise in a horizontal transverse plane, with some irregularity of direction and columnar arrangement. A long, heavy dendrite extends from each end of the cell; the axon extends transversely from the midpoint of the cell body. The dendritic processes receive numerous boutons. On sectioning the trapezoid body experimentally all of these boutons degenerate; all of the nerve cells of the medial dorsal olive show retrograde degeneration following section of the lateral lemniscus. It would appear that the main function of the nucleus is the condensing and forwarding of the nerve impulses of the main afferent auditory pathway. This would require the maintaining as distinct, in some way not currently understood, multiple messages forwarded over single nerve fibers, as the stated process of convergence does not appear to blunt the capacity for frequency discrimination or to cause loss of any integration

Figure 26A. Lower-power view of right dorsal olivary complex to show the general arrangement of the components. (Facial nucleus is rounded area at right upper composed of large neurons.) Medial dorsal olivary nucleus is seen as a vertical column at lower left (two arrows) with its lower portion bent to right. Lateral dorsal olivary nucleus is a not-too-cellular, rounded cell cluster below the facial nucleus (arrow). Divers cells scattered in surrounding region are periolivary and comprise a portion of the field referred to inclusively as the trapezoid nucleus.

Figure 26B. Higher power of a portion of a (left) medial dorsal olivary nucleus showing the bipolar fusiform character of the cells. Granularity of some of the intercellular tissue is unexplained as to origin; some if it represents lipochrome as wear-and-tear pigment.

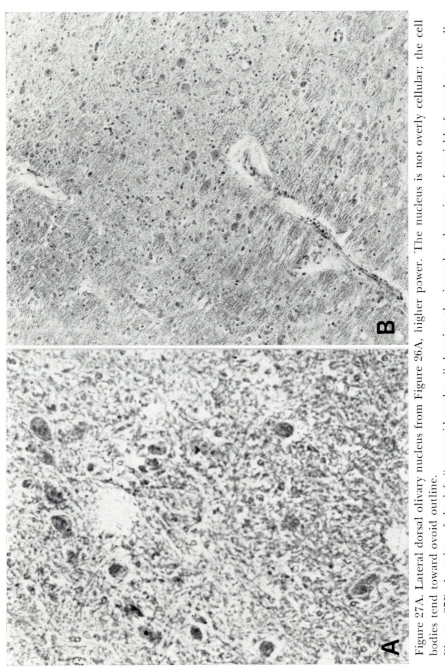

Figure 27A. Lateral dorsal olivary nucleus from Figure 26A, higher power. The cell bodies tend toward ovoid outline.

Figures 27B. A region of the left "trapezoid nucleus," showing the irregular clustering of variably formed nerve cells. Fibers of the trapezoid body are seen sweeping across especially the lower left portion of the field.

achieved within the cochlear nucleus. Orientation within the medial dorsal olive could be achieved by virtue of positional organization of the synaptic terminals.

The lateral dorsal olivary nucleus lies just lateral to the dorsal portion of the medial dorsal olivary nucleus in the angle formed by the latter and the facial nucleus. In the human the lateral dorsal olive is roughly ovoid to cylindrical; in transverse sections it appears as a comparatively sparse and inconstant cluster of medium-sized to large, round to ovoid plump nerve cells showing no particular pattern of arrangement. The cells possess scant dendrites; the cytoplasm shows some fine Nissl substance.

Certain periolivary cell clusters and the trapezoid nucleus are comparatively distinct in some lower animals as in the cat, but in the human they are insufficiently organized for recognition (Olszewski and Baxter, 1954). They may be referred to collectively as periolivary cells, or as the trapezoid nucleus, providing the latter term implies only a field. The trapezoid nucleus appears to be represented less on the dorsal side of the dorsal olivary nuclei than in the three other directions. It is best developed in relation to the caudal half of the medial dorsal olive. There is an irregular and inconstant tendency toward gathering of the trapezoid nucleus into small clusters. The appearance of the cells is essentially that of the cells of the lateral dorsal olivary nucleus, with the appearance of a few multipolar forms (Olszewski and Baxter, 1954).

The nuclei of the lateral lemniscus (Olszewski and Baxter, 1954) are essentially two—ventral and dorsal. The former is roughly cylindrical; it lies lateral to the cranial aspect of the medial dorsal olivary nucleus. Bordered by the gathering fibers of the lateral lemniscus, the nucleus extends cranialward for a distance of about 8 mm. The nerve cells of the nucleus are medium in size, round to ovoid, sometimes multipolar, distributed comparatively loosely. The dorsal nucleus is a small, irregular and inconstant cluster of cells, sometimes multicentric, lying in the lateral lemniscus where the latter swings dorsolaterally into the lateral wall of the midbrain. Its component cells resemble those of the ventral nucleus.

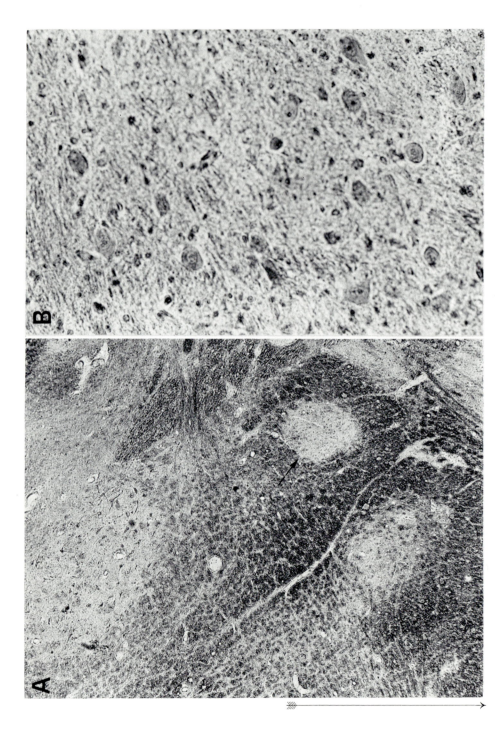

The Inferior Colliculus

The inferior colliculi (Geniec and Morest, 1971; Olszewski and Baxter, 1954) are two rounded elevations forming the caudal half of the mesencephalic tectal plate. They extend from the level of the oral extremity of the anterior medullary velum to the transitional zone which separates the inferior from the superior colliculi. Each inferior colliculus exhibits a dorsal, superficial cortex, a central nucleus and pericollicular tegmentum (Geniec and Morest, 1971).

The central nucleus is oval on cross section; it lies with its long axis directed obliquely, dorsomedially. Fibers of the lateral lemniscus, extending to the cortex dorsally and to the pericollicular tegmentum ventrally, form a capsule about the ventrolateral pole of the central nucleus. The dorsomedial extremity of the brachium of the inferior colliculus appears adjoining the rostrolateral aspect of the central nucleus. Dorsomedially, the central nuclei approach one another dorsal to the central gray matter of the cerebral aqueduct, and in this region the distinction between the collicular and aqueductal gray matter may be difficult. In the oral portion of the inferior colliculus this dorsal region is traversed by commissural fibers; the latter, however, are most numerous in the transition zone between inferior and superior colliculi.

The cortex of the inferior colliculus separates the central nucleus dorsally and caudally from the surface of the collicular convexity. The peri-collicular tegmentum separates the central nucleus from the superior colliculus, from the lateral surface of the tectum, and from the underlying region of the midbrain tegmentum.

Microscopically, the central nucleus is quite cellular, and this impression is heightened by the presence of numerous glial cells, many of which are satellitic. The nerve cells vary considerably in

---

Figure 28A. Low power view, Weil's myelin stain, of dorsal olivary complex slightly rostral to section of Figure 26A. The ventral nucleus (arrow) of the lateral lemniscus appears as a relatively pale area surrounded by dark-staining fibers of the lateral lemniscus.

Figure 28B. Higher power view of the nucleus showing not-too-densely arranged ovoid nerve cells.

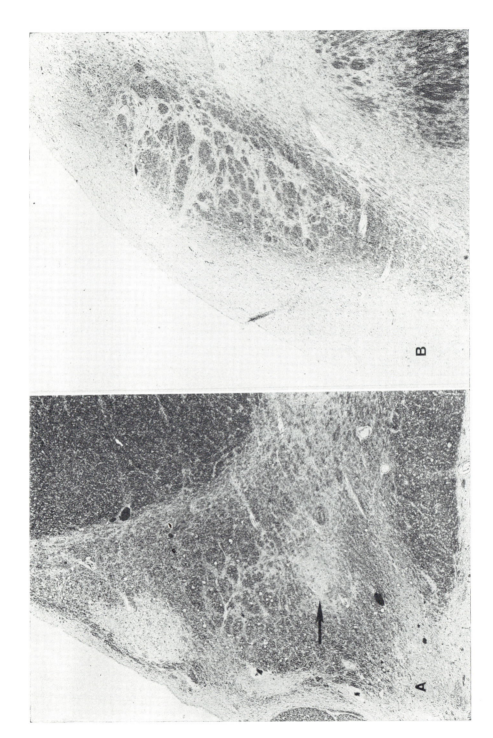

size and shape, exhibiting fusiform, triangular and ovoid out-lines, the types intermingled without regionalization. Especially in the caudal portion of the central nucleus the cells tend toward arrangement in columns parallel with the incoming fibers of the lateral lemniscus, and the long axes of the cell bodies are directed with the same linearity. This appearance is emphasized by the columnation of accompanying glial cells, especially if the latter are increased in number, and capillaries show the same directional character.

In Golgi preparations, this linear feature is accentuated by the structure of the dendrites, revealing a well-developed lamina-tion. The laminae tend to diverge as they extend dorsomedially from the ventrolateral region of the central nucleus, reconverging on approaching the dorsomedial region. In the rostral portion of the central nucleus the fiber pattern becomes more complex and the nerve cells are arranged in a more haphazard manner. The neurons of the central nucleus have been classed on the basis of shape of dendritic field; the five recognized types are small and large disc-shaped and small, medium and large stellate (Geniec and Morest, 1971). A functional significance of differences in in-dividual cell structure is not apparent.

The cortex is a thin strip of nerve cells of different types and sizes; it is less cellular than the central nucleus. Some degree of layering has been observed (Geniec and Morest, 1971); this ap-pears less clear and uniform than in the central nucleus. Four layers are recognized, but the more superficial ones attenuate caudally and eventually disappear. A fifth layer may be dis-tinguished anteromedially. The cells of the more superficial zone tend to be fusiform with larger, multipolar neurons found more deeply. These latter cells, especially, are equipped by position and structure for integrative monitoring of impulses to and from the

Figure 29A. An aggregated portion of the dorsal nucleus (arrow) of the left lateral lemniscus lies within the lemniscus; the latter is turning up toward the inferior colliculus.

Figure 29B. Further, less-clearly-aggregated portion of the dorsal nucleus of the left lateral lemniscus within the latter as it extends up toward the in-ferior colliculus. Weil's myelin stain.

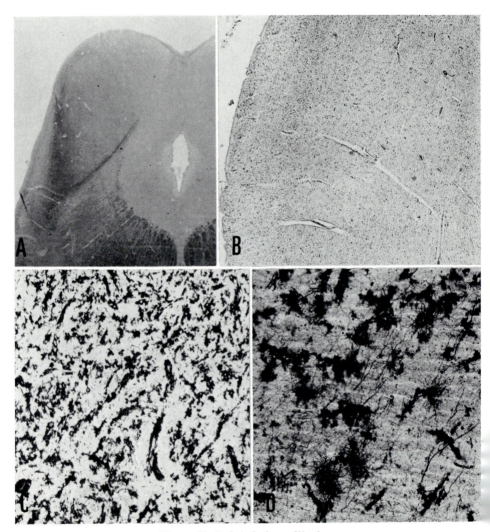

Figure 30. Left inferior colliculus.
Figure 30A. Weil's myelin stain showing lateral lemniscus forming a capsule about the central nucleus, extending upward from ventrolateral pole.
Figure 30B. Cortex and major substance of the central nucleus as seen in transverse section. The incoming fibers of the lateral lemniscus produce an appearance of fine striation from lower left to upper right.
Figure 30 C,D. Golgi preparation. Figure 30C. A laminated structure is apparent, the laminae extending from ventrolateral (lower left) to dorsomedial (upper right). Figure 30D. Higher power view showing the polarized arrangement of the dendritic pattern in same direction.

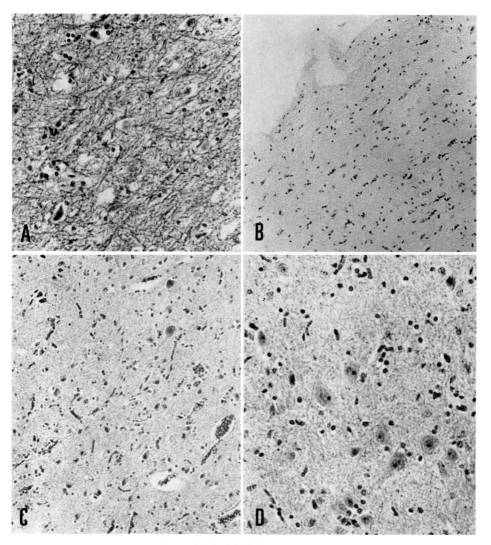

Figure 31. Left inferior colliculus.

Figure 31A. Bodian preparation of the dorsomedial and superior portion showing the crossing of fibers of the lateral lemniscus, extending from lower left (ventrolateral) to upper right (dorsomedial), with horizontal transverse fibers of the commissure.

Figure 31B. Fusiform cells of the cortex.

Figure 31C. The laminated structure of the central nucleus is shown with orientation from ventrolateral to dorsomedial (lower left to upper right).

Figure 31D. Nerve cells of the central nucleus, varying in size and appearing in ovoid, triangular and fusiform shapes. Glial cells are plentiful.

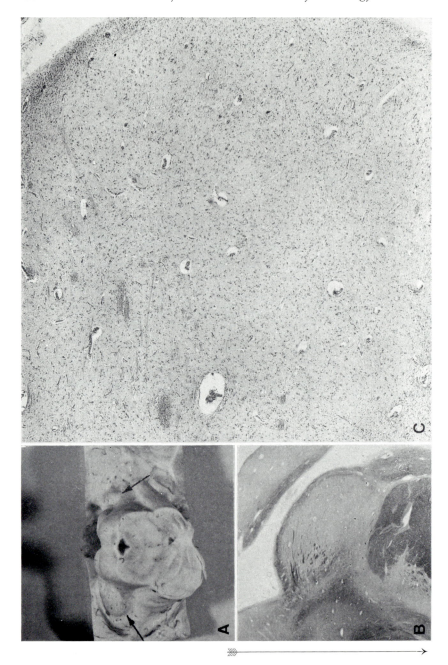

central nucleus (Geniec and Morest, 1971).

The peri-collicular tegmentum (Geniec and Morest, 1971) is a thin layer of cells whose reported extent was noted previously. It is not universally recognized as a separate structure (Olszewski and Baxter, 1954). Subdivisional nuclei and zones have been described with the consideration that the neuronal groups may provide for interactions of the auditory and somatic sensory pathways (Geniec and Morest, 1971).

The inferior colliculus is considered to participate in the transmission of afferent auditory impulses to the medial geniculate bodies, in the integration of ascending and descending auditory pathways, and in the elaboration of acoustic reflexes (Geniec and Morest, 1971). Only deep lesions of the inferior colliculus, presumably involving the central nucleus, produced gross hearing losses in experimental animals (von Bechterew, 1895, quoted by Geniec and Morest, 1971). Acoustically-evoked responses in the cat have been found limited to the central nucleus (Massopust and Ordy, 1962). Electrical stimulation of the surface of the inferior colliculus of a human produced no conscious sensation (Simmons, Mongeon, Lewis and Huntington, 1964). Following bilateral section of the brachium of the inferior colliculus in the cat, the subjects could not localize sound. Unilateral section resulted in a large transient loss of localizing ability with some permanent impairment (Strominger and Oesterreich, 1970).

Figure 32. Right medial geniculate body.

Figure 32A. There was old infarction of the middle cerebral artery region of supply with destruction of the auditory area along with other tissues (see Figure 82). Descending degeneration of the pyramidal tract has occurred. The inferior colliculi appear normal. The lateral division of the right medial geniculate body is atrophic, leaving unaltered the medial nuclear division (arrow) compared with the left medial geniculate (arrow).

Figure 32B. Transverse section of normal medial geniculate body, Weil's myelin stain, appearing centrally as an ovoid structure; a few fibers of the brachium of the inferior colliculus are seen at the upper left pole.

Figure 32C. Low power of the medial geniculate. The slightly relatively pale, irregularly round region occupying roughly the ventromedial (lower left) one fourth of the field represents the medial division; the principal division is the remaining tissue, extending around the medial division in an outline earning the term *geniculate.*

The Medial Geniculate Body

The medial geniculate body appears as a small rounded elevation on the posterior aspect of each thalamus. The greatest dimension is anteroposterior. Each medial geniculate body lies at the termination of the brachium of the inferior colliculus; it extends forward beyond roughly one third of the lateral geniculate body.

Histologically, the medial geniculate body exhibits considerable heterogeneity of neuronal type, fiber architecture and afferent telodendria (Morest, 1964). Especially as seen in Nissl preparations (Rose and Galambos, 1952), the medial geniculate presents a ventromedial division, the pars magnocellularis, composed of comparatively large, loosely-arranged nerve cells, and a principal division, the relatively small-celled, more densely-populated pars parvocellularis, a reniform structure curved in frontal as well as horizontal planes; it extends around the pars magnocellularis with its convexity directed laterally, forming the free surface of the medial geniculate (the latter term is well-deserved). A hilus is occupied by fibers of the brachium of the inferior colliculus and the auditory radiation as they enter or leave the nuclear center.

In the medial geniculate body, the usual two basic types of neurons are recognized—Golgi type I with long projecting axons and type II with short axons. The small type II neurons are thought to have an inhibitory effect (Morest, 1971).

In the cat, on the basis of dendritic branching pattern, it has been proposed to divide the pars principalis into dorsal and ventral portions; the basis for such a distinction was depicted some years ago, although without recognition (Morest, 1964; Monakow, 1882, quoted by Morest, 1964). The recognized types of dendritic structure are two in number—radiate, showing dichotomous branching and found in the dorsal division, and tufted, appearing in the ventral division (Morest, 1964). The dorsal division is relatively pale-staining in myelin preparations. The ventral division appears rich in myelinated fibers. This division presents a more tightly-woven intrinsic afferent fiber plexus than the dorsal division does. There is a laminar arrangement of the neurons of the ventral division, the laminae sweeping from ventromedial to dorsolateral in a curved pattern, forming diagonal to vertical cell columns (Morest, 1964, 1965) (*see* Figures 33 A & B).

The pars principalis appears to be the sole auditory portion of the medial geniculate. The magnocellular part does not send fibers to the auditory cortex (Whitfield, 1967), nor can single unit activity be recorded (Rose and Galambos, 1952). This division does not undergo retrograde degeneration when the auditory cortex is destroyed. The magnocellular division may be the site for convergence of a number of fiber systems (Goldberg and Moore, 1967) (*see* Figures 34 A & B).

The ventral division of the principal nucleus is said to project to the primary auditory area and to serve as the terminus for fibers from the inferior colliculus (Rasmussen, 1964). The dorsal division is considered to have a multiplicity of dissimilar connections, largely undetermined, in contrast to the relatively homogeneous input of the ventral division, and its cortical projection may represent more than one sensory modality (Morest, 1964). The dorsal division may be seen to undergo retrograde degeneration following destruction of the region of the brain supplied by the middle cerebral artery, including the superior temporal convolution. This suggests that the dorsal division of the pars principalis projects within the stated region but does not identify further the point or points of termination (*see* Figure 35).

Further parcellation of the dorsal and ventral divisions into nuclear subgroups has been made in the cat (Morest, 1964). This feature, together with applicability to the human, invites further evaluation (*see* Figure 36).

The Auditory Cortex

The position and extent of the auditory cortex cannot be stated unequivocally (Whitfield, 1967). This becomes increasingly problematic the further one proceeds from an apparent primary center into surrounding, possibly associational, regions. Much of the available information is concerning lower animals, not necessarily offering reliable application to the human. Many variables are encountered. The obliquely extending anterior transverse temporal gyrus (of Heschl) is considered to represent the primary

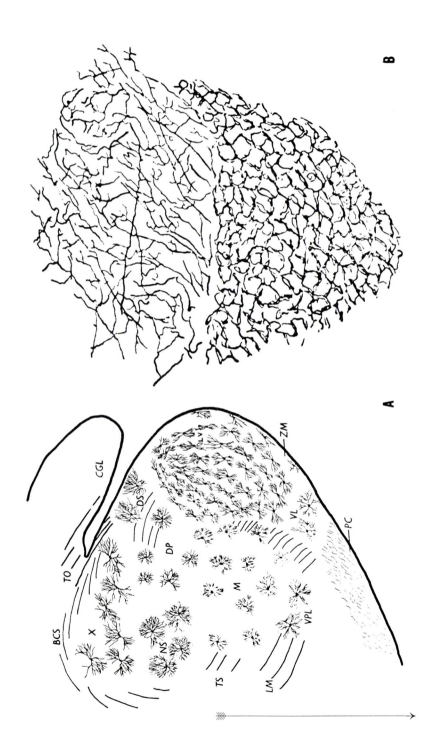

auditory projection field, Brodmann's area 41 (Truex and Carpenter, 1969). This area delineation traditionally does not depict the floor of the Sylvian fissure. The adjacent cortex is referred to as area 42, largely an associational area. Area 22, occupying a certain adjacent portion of the superior temporal gyrus, is thought to receive fibers from areas 41 and 42 and to have connections with regions of the occipital, parietal and insular cortex. A variable is encountered in the notable difference observed in the convolutional pattern of the transverse temporal gyri as to number, outline and relative proportions of the convolutions (*see* Figure 37).

Histologically, the primary auditory cortex is somewhat thick; it is composed of small nerve cells, being of the granular type referred to as koniocortex (Truex and Carpenter, 1969). The cells are concentrated somewhat in two bands as in the primary visual area, a similarity that possibly is not without significance. A striking difference is encountered, however, in an individually characteristic columnation perpendicular to the pial surface. In the examples studied thus far the anterior transverse gyrus has shown this cellular pattern throughout its length; the posterior transverse gyrus has not exhibited such a pattern except for skip areas in those cases in which the more posterior column is relatively large. The bearing of this observation on the delineation of the primary auditory cortex is evident; its validity, however, depends on the significance of cellular architecture in relation to the functional outlining of the primary sensory area. Except as just mentioned, the posterior transverse convolution is of the parietal type showing the usual six-layered arrangement of differ-

---

Figure 33A. Schematic drawing of transverse section of right medial geniculate body, Golgi preparation. (M) Medial nucleus. The neurons of the dorsal portion (DP) of the pars lateralis have a radiate dendritic pattern while those of the ventral division (VL) are tufted. There is a laminar arrangement of the neurons of the ventral division, the laminae sweeping from ventromedial to dorsolateral in a curved pattern and forming diagonal to vertical cell columns. After Morest, *J. Anat, 98*:611, 1964.

Figure 33B. Schematic drawing of lateral division of medial geniculate body. Golgi preparation happened to delineate the intrinsic afferent fiber plexus. The ventral division appears to show a more dense pattern than the dorsal division does. After Morest, *J. Anat, 98*:611, 1964.

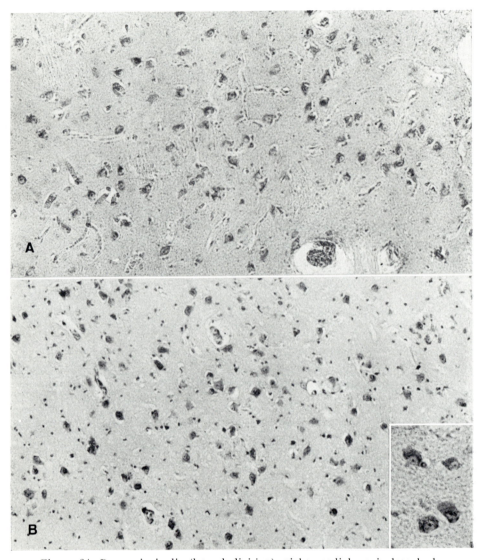

Figure 34. Pars principalis (lateral division), right medial geniculate body, cresyl violet.

Figure 34A. Dorsal division. Distribution of cells is haphazard.

Figure 34B. Ventral division. Some degree of cell columnation is apparent even in the Nissl preparation, especially in the lower portion of the illustration, the columns extending diagonally upward to the right. Inset: Cells from ventral division showing three Golgi type I cells (larger) and one type II cell (smaller).

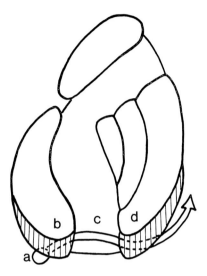

Figure 35. Schematic drawing of auditory radiation. (a) Medial geniculate body; curving double-lined arrow represents auditory radiation. (b) Pulvinar. (c) Posterior limb of internal capsule. (d) Lenticular nucleus. Modified, after Truex and Carpenter, *Human Neuroanatomy*, Ed. VI, Williams and Wilkins, 1969.

ent cell types with the appearance of some large pyramidal cells in layer III. This corresponds to earlier report of the structure of area 42 (Truex and Carpenter, 1969).

Electron microscopic studies have shown the auditory cortex to be densely packed with nerve cells and their processes and neuroglial elements. Only very small spaces separate the plasma membranes of the different cellular elements; the extracellular volume of the auditory cortex cannot be appreciable (de Lorenzo, 1960b).

Consequent to the bilateral representation of hearing at the cortical level, hemispherectomy has no noteworthy effect upon hearing as judged by the pure tone audiogram (Dix and Hood, 1973). The bilateral ablation of the auditory cortex in the cat does not alter the pure tone threshold of hearing (Neff, 1960). Destruction of the auditory cortex should theoreticaly result in

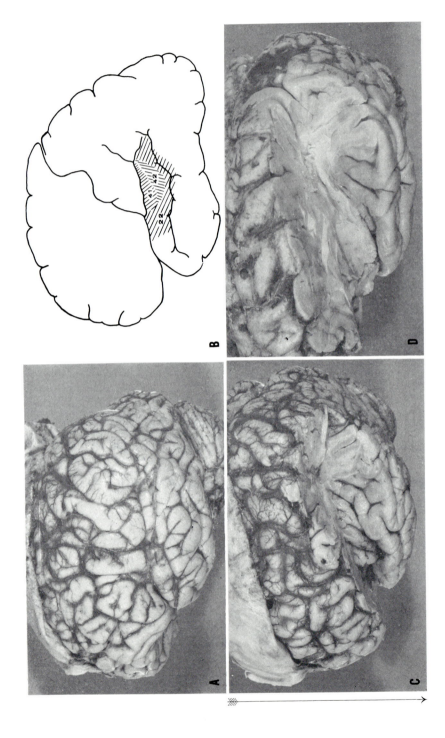

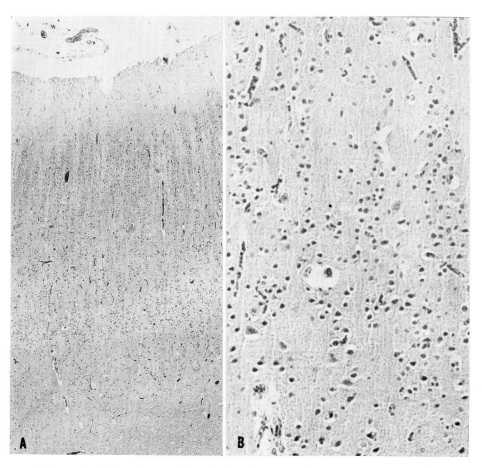

Figure 37. Microphotographs of the primary auditory cortex with higher magnification (Figure 37B) of a field in lower left center of Figure 37A, lower power. Columnation transverse to the surface is shown. The cells are somewhat uniformly small (koniocortex) with a few interspersed larger cells.

Figure 36. Gross delineation of auditory cortex.

Figure 36A. Lateral and slightly superior view of brain.

Figure 36B. The same. Drawing shows the main fissures for comparative orientation and indicates the auditory areas according to Brodmann.

Figures 36C and D. Two views of the exposed superior temporal gyrus illustrating variation in size and arrangement of the transverse gyri.

diminished acuity; however, this is not borne out in most practical testing circumstances (Minckler, 1972). Well-documented, unequivocally-measured reduction in auditory sensitivity with a clearly demonstrated central nervous system lesion and no demonstrable peripheral lesion has not been reported (Jerger, Weikers, Sharbrough *et al.*, 1969).* Lesions of especially the posterior portion of area 22, unilateral dominant hemisphere or bilateral, are thought to produce receptive or sensory aphasia. It is difficult, however, to establish the lesions that result in different forms of aphasia (Truex and Carpenter, 1969). Areas 41, 42 and 22 are not established well enough to justify their consideration as discrete functional zones (Schuknecht, 1974). The general weight of evidence supports the view that the auditory cortex is concerned not with the perception of frequency and intensity, but rather with the recognition of temporal patterns (Whitfield, 1967). It would appear that in cases of sensorineural hearing loss the value of the histopathologic study of the primary auditory region will be in relation to a somewhat broad structural documentation of clinically-established integrative deficits.

Afferent Projections and Connections

Most available information regarding the central auditory pathway is based on studies in lower animals, not necessarily applicable to the human (Barnes, Magoun and Ranson, 1943). The structure of the pathway is complex, and many details remain uncertain or subject to difference of opinion. The present discussion is intended as a simple and basic account, and further, must be regarded as tentative.

The fiber tracts of the auditory pathway receive contributions from a number of intercalated sources; the existence of reflex connections and integrative complexes appears well-established.

The central projection of the cochlear nuclear complex is effected by three striae—dorsal (Monakow), intermediate (Held) and ventral (trapezoid body). Only the latter is visible in non-

---

*Certain lesions of the cochlear nuclei would need to be excluded from this generalization.

pathologic specimens; it is larger in bulk than the other two bundles combined. Its fibers are relatively large and heavily myelinated while the fibers of the dorsal and intermediate striae are comparatively fine; this difference suggests the existence of faster and slower-conducting fiber systems (Barnes, Magoun and Ranson, 1943).

The dorsal acoustic stria represents the central projection of the dorsal cochlear nucleus. A thin bundle, it is the least of the striae. Its fibers pass medialward over the restiform body, then turn somewhat ventrally and cross the midline ventral to the median longitudinal fasciculus to join the medial part of the contralateral lateral lemniscus (Osen, 1972; Stotler, 1953; Truex and Carpenter, 1969; Whitfield, 1967). Central termination has been variably stated as being (1) the central nucleus of the inferior colliculus (a) without added synapse (Barnes, Magoun and Ranson, 1943), (b) with the addition of the nuclei of the lateral lemniscus (Stotler, 1953) and (2) satellitic dorsal olivary cell groups (Fernandez and Karapas, 1967). Section of the lateral lemniscus (cat) produced retrograde degeneration of the cells of the contralateral dorsal cochlear nucleus, but none in the ventral cochlear nucleus (synapse intervening in the dorsal olivary nuclei) (Osen, 1972); the latter was affected when the trapezoid body was cut. These features of contralateral projection and the apparent limitation of number of synapses are individually peculiar to the dorsal cochlear nucleus; they suggest a comparatively primitive type of auditory function.

The intermediate acoustic stria appears to arise from the inferior portion of the inferior ventral cochlear nucleus where the octopoid cells are found (Osen, 1969a). The fibers of this stria pass centrally along with those of the ventral acoustic stria in the trapezoid body (Stotler, 1953); the fibers terminate on satellitic dorsal olivary cells (Fernandez and Karapas, 1967). (Specific cell clusters are identified in the cat, but not in the human.)

The ventral acoustic stria emanates from the bulk of the ventral cochlear nucleus. The course and termination of processes of certain of the large types of cells is uncertain. On a basis of population density and proportion, as well as potential application of experimental work in the cat, it appears that the main source is the spheroid cells (Dublin, 1974; Osen, 1969a). The trapezoid body sweeps ventromedially in a gentle arc beneath the restiform body to supply the homolateral dendrites of the fusiform cells of the medial dorsal olivary nucleus, i.e. if from the right cochlear nucleus, the right-sided dendrites (Stotler, 1953; Strominger and Strominger, 1971). This involves a considerable reduction in units of the pathway and is effected with terminal boutons.

This division of the pathway into crossed and uncrossed units produces the first level of bilateral audition. Each medial dorsal olive is thought to send fibers superiorward on the same side (Stotler, 1953).

The lateral dorsal olivary nucleus is regressive in man. It is presumably supplied with fibers from the ventral cochlear nucleus of the same side. Bilateral representation is achieved by crossing of a roughly equal portion of the ascending fibers as they leave the nucleus and project superiorward (Stotler, 1953).

The crossed division of the olivo-cochlear bundle is thought to arise in cells of the periolivary region (trapezoid nuclear field); otherwise the course and termination of fibers leaving this nuclear region is unknown (Stotler, 1953).

The ventral nucleus of the lateral lemniscus appears to contribute fibers to the lemniscus, the latter, at its origin, margining the nucleus. This nucleus sends some commissural fibers to the corresponding nucleus of the opposite side and some to the adjacent reticular formation (Stotler, 1953).

The lateral lemniscus is the main passage from the dorsal olive to the inferior colliculus. Few if any fibers extend directly in the lateral lemniscus from the ventral cochlear nucleus. The main source of the lemniscus, the axons of the fusiform cells of the medial dorsal olive, project transversely from the cell bodies. It is remarkable that complex details of frequency as well as those of modifying or integrating impulses supplied to the spheroid cells of the ventral cochlear nucleus, can be maintained in proper order while passing over so reduced a number of nerve fibers. All cells of the medial dorsal olive react to destruction of the inferior colliculus: that is, no fibers are projected from the medial dorsal olive to the reticular formation or to other brain stem nuclei

(Stotler, 1953). This lends possible support to the previously-stated concept that the spheroid cells supplying the medial dorsal olive are essentially the second-order neurons of the main afferent auditory pathway while the other large neurons could engage more in associational and/or reflex activity.

The lateral lemniscus extends superiorly and gradually dorsolaterally toward the inferolateral aspect of the inferior colliculus; it terminates almost entirely in the central nucleus, supplying all parts of the nucleus (Osen, 1972; Stotler, 1953). A few fibers end in the caudal sector of the external nucleus (cortex) (cat and squirrel monkey) (Goldberg and Moore, 1967).

No fibers from the ventral cochlear nucleus reach the inferior colliculus directly; all have synapsed at least once enroute (Rasmussen, 1946; Stotler, 1953). The proportion of fibers of the lateral lemniscus retaining frequency specificity diminishes passing upward in the brain stem: for example, there is a progressively increasing number of fibers of collateral import.

Each inferior colliculus connects with its opposite by means of the commissure. These fibers appear to have ipsilateral pathway origin; it is a general rule that pathways which have crossed at lower levels do not cross back again. Some fibers from the inferior colliculus reach the superior colliculus, apparently supplying cells contributing to tectobulbar and tectospinal tracts. Most fibers from the inferior colliculus extend in the main afferent auditory pathway through the brachium of the inferior colliculus to the medial geniculate body. No lemniscal fibers reach the medial geniculate body directly; a fiber bundle (not synapsing in the inferior colliculus) extending in the brachium appears to be of spinal origin, is nonauditory, and terminates in the medial part of the magnocellular division.

From the medial geniculate the final link of the afferent auditory pathway extends forward and lateralward beneath the pulvinar of the thalamus, lateralward through the posterior extremity of the posterior limb of the internal capsule, beneath the posterior margin of the putamen, and turns upward and forward in the auditory radiation (Fig. 35) to reach the primary auditory cortex. Most fibers of the radiation are thought to project to area 41, a few extending to area 42.

The Efferent Pathway

There is a descending conduction system paralleling the afferent auditory pathway from the cortex to the cochlea (Rasmussen, 1960). This provides a feedback mechanism of integration and control. Centers such as the cochlear nuclei and inferior colliculi receive fibers descending from higher levels. Stimulation at various points along the descending pathway will produce a diminution of response to clicks in the cochlear nucleus (Comis and Whitfield, 1967).

An outstanding efferent system is that which includes the olivocochlear bundle (Rasmussen, 1946). This bundle consists of a crossed component and a homolateral component, the former possessing about four times the number of fibers found in the latter. On the basis of experimental work in the cat it is thought that the crossed division arises in the satellitic dorsal olivary field; this is not discretely organized in the human (Olszewski and Baxter, 1954). The homolateral portion originates from the lateral dorsal olive (Rasmussen, 1960). The crossed bundle passes dorsally to cross the midline just beneath the abducens nucleus; it is joined by the homolateral portion lateral to the outgoing facial root. Some fibers of the olivocochlear bundle extend through the vestibular nerve to supply the cochlear nucleus. The remaining fibers leave the brain stem in company with the vestibular nerve between its superior and inferior divisions. They extend through the vestibulocochlear anastomosis to join the cochlear nerve and enter the spiral canal of the modiolus where they form the intraganglionic spiral bundle. Their further course was described previously.

Stimulation of the olivocochlear bundle results in suppression of auditory nerve activity (Galambos, 1956). It has been observed, however, that sectioning of the crossed olivocochlear bundle, where stimulation of the bundle before sectioning produced suppression of action potential, had no effect on adaptation or round window-recorded action potential in response to successive auditory stimuli (Dayal, 1972). Similarly, on transecting the crossed olivocochlear bundle, the pure tone threshold was not altered (Igarashi, Alford, Nakai and Gordon, 1972).

Efferent nerve fibers and endings are, as a general class, cholinesterase positive (Gacek, Nomura and Balogh, 1965; Rasmussen, 1964, 1967; Schuknecht, Churchill and Doran, 1959).

Blood Supply

The basilar artery is formed by the junction of the two vertebrals; it divides to give rise to the posterior cerebral arteries. The brain stem is supplied by the vertebral-basilar system (Gillilan, 1964). The posterior inferior cerebellar arteries arise from the vertebrals while the superior and anterior inferior cerebellar arteries and small pontine branches most often are contributed by the basilar. The superior cerebellar artery is more constant in origin and pattern than are the others. Vertebral-basilar tributaries are of two main types—superficial, running on the surface of the brain stem, and penetrating or intrinsic (Gillilan, 1964). The latter tend to arise in clusters from the concealed surfaces of the parent superficial vessels and extend transversely into the brain stem. They are comparatively small, many of them being of arteriolar caliber. They fall into four major zones—median (midline), paramedian, lateral and dorsal. The superficial arteries vary considerably in course and pattern; the intrinsic vessels are more constant. Accordingly, the regions or outlines of vascular brain stem lesions, reflecting on categorization of syndromes, are better related to the intrinsic vascular pattern than to the superficial. It is especially difficult to separate reliably the territories of the two inferior cerebellar arteries. Further, anastomosis is common between the two inferior cerebellar arteries on the surface of the cerebellum. The cerebral and cerebellar hemispheres have a pial arteriolar plexus, but none is found on the surface of the brain stem.

The region of the cochlear nuclear complex and some adjoining portions of the eighth nerve and of pons and medulla are supplied by branches of the anterior inferior cerebellar artery (Adams, 1943) (inferolateral pontine region [Gillilan, 1964]). Symptoms of occlusion of this vessel (or regional vessels) include tinnitus, ipsilateral total nerve deafness and slight impairment of hearing on the opposite side (Adams, 1943), implicating involvement of dorsal olivary, trapezoid and/or lateral lemniscal elements serving the pathway of contralateral origin.

The inferior colliculus is supplied in most cases by the superior cerebellar artery through one or several rami; on occasion, twigs may arise from the posterior cerebral artery. The central nucleus is supplied by the lateral arterial system, the vessels entering the nucleus among the afferent fiber bundles. The dorsolateral half of the medial geniculate body receives penetrating arteries of the dorsal arterial group that arise from the posterior cerebral.

The auditory radiation and cortex are supplied by ganglionic and cortical branches of the middle cerebral artery.

SOME MISCELLANEOUS PRINCIPLES

The Tonotopic Frequency Scale

There appears to be a tonotopic frequency gradient throughout the afferent auditory pathway; this is well-supported as far as the inferior colliculus.

In the organ of Corti high frequencies are represented at the base with progression to low frequencies at the apex. In the cat a nearly linear spatial distribution exists, on the organ of Corti, of the logarithmic frequency scale in the range of 500 to 32,000 cps (Schuknecht, 1960). The frequency scale is similarly represented in the spiral ganglion. The application of this general principle to the human cochlea is indicated by the demonstration of lesions of the basal turn in the high-frequency hearing loss (Guild, 1932, 1937; Schuknecht, 1960, 1964).

Tonotopic structure has been demonstrated in the cochlear nucleus of lower animals. Anatomically, primary afferent cochlear nerve fibers were found to be distributed with a range from low frequency ventrolateral to high frequency dorsomedial (Sando, 1965; van Noort, 1969). Physiologically, a tonotopic scale has been demonstrated for each of the three cochlear nuclear subdivisions separately, low frequencies ventral to high frequencies dorsal (Rose, Galambos and Hughes, 1960). This was done by locating a series of *best frequencies* with the exploring electrode. (The *best frequency* is the frequency at which a given unit is activated at an intensity at which other frequencies are ineffective.)

A similar tonotopic pattern appears to exist in the human, high frequencies dorsal to low frequencies ventral. This is more susceptible to demonstration in the ventral nucleus than in the dorsal subdivision, considering the thinness of the latter in the human. In certain conditions in which there is a high-tone hearing loss of central or so-called nuclear type with maximal loss at around 2,000 to 4,000 cps, if the process is sufficiently moderate so as to result in cell injury of a certain portion of the ventral nucleus rather than in its complete destruction, a zone of alteration will be found in the dorsal portion of the ventral nucleus (especially clearly seen in the superior subdivision) although sparing the dorsalmost extremity (Dublin, 1974).

Tonotopicity in the cochlear nucleus would appear to be in relation to the spheroid cells. Considerably more study is needed for a proper evaluation of the general problem; however, data available to date suggests that the tonotopic frequency scale on the ventral cochlear nucleus corresponds to the straight-line logarithmic function of frequency. The distribution of spheroid cells in the inferior ventral nucleus and the converging curvature of the dorsalmost and ventralmost margins of the ventral nuclear subdivisions, affecting total numbers of cells in ventrodorsally progressive cross-section strata, invite further evaluation of the structural basis of frequency.

The quality of frequency as it emerges from the cochlear nucleus appears to rest not upon any intrinsic feature of the nucleus, but upon the frequency character of the impulse presented to the nucleus, requiring only to be preserved according to the pointwise anatomic correspondence of cochlear nucleus to cochlea. Modification of the impulse occurring within the nucleus apparently is integrative, not affecting frequency per se.

The medial dorsal olivary nucleus has shown a tonotopic frequency gradient under experimental conditions. This nucleus is especially well-developed in the dog, providing a favorable experimental subject. The gradient is high frequency ventral to low frequency dorsal, the arrangement being opposite to that in the cochlear nucleus. Maximum in cps was found to be 11,800 (Goldberg and Brown, 1968), in keeping with the range expected from spheroid cells.

The trapezoid nuclear field and the nuclei of the lateral lemniscus offer little opportunity for evaluation of tonotopicity; they appear, in any event, to be concerned with factors other than the frequency scale.

A tonotopic frequency gradient has been demonstrated in the central nucleus of the inferior colliculus (cat), progressing from low to high frequencies in a ventral, oral and medial direction (Rose, Grenwood, Goldberg and Hind, 1963); such direction is perpendicular to the cellular laminae of the central nucleus; the lamination may well bear a relation to the tonotopic frequency pattern. In the cortex, a high to low frequency was found in a direction opposite to that in the central nucleus; these latter results were considered less certain. The surgically-exposed pial surface of the human inferior colliculus was found insensitive to stimulation (Simmons, Mongeon, Lewis and Huntington, 1964).

The question of tonotopicity in the medial geniculate body is subject to variance of opinion and invites clarification. Evidence in support of such tonotopicity includes the laminar structure of the ventral division. Experimental stimulation of the basal turn of the cochlea was effective only in the medial portion of the pars principalis while the stimulation of apical fibers was effective only laterally, suggesting a transverse tonotopic frequency gradient (Rose and Woolsey, 1958). The direction of tonotopic progression, if arranged transverse to the laminae, would be from dorsomedial to ventrolateral.

The columnation observed in the auditory cortex similarly suggests a relation to the frequency scale. On experimental stimulation (cat) of small groups of cochlear nerve fibers, a point-to-point projection to specific portions of the auditory cortex was found. A secondary system with opposite polarity of the frequency gradient was observed (Woolsey and Walzl, 1942). In the monkey a corresponding auditory area was found within the sylvian fissure on the dorsal aspect of the temporal lobe, with higher frequencies posteromedial and lower frequencies anterolateral. Comparability with the anterior transverse temporal gyrus in the human is apparent. On the basis of presently available information, however, a tonotopic frequency pattern cannot be considered established in the human. It is suggested that this cortical region is concerned, rather, with the discrimination of time-dependent signals (sequential patterns) (Whitfield, 1967).

Zonal Vulnerability of the Ventral Cochlear Nucleus

The basal turn of the cochlea displays a characteristic susceptibility to injury by various pathogenic factors. The aforementioned finding of cell degeneration in a certain zone of the ventral cochlear nucleus indicates that this structure also exhibits a topistic pattern of vulnerability (Dublin, 1974). This is seen characteristically in cases involving anoxia. The gradient of susceptibility, however, does not pertain to the dorsal cochlear nucleus, which in any event is too thin and sparse to permit much in the way of stratified analysis. The view formerly advanced that injury of the dorsal cochlear nucleus is responsible for high-tone hearing loss consequent to factors such as the high rate of metabolism, rich capillary vascularity and high-frequency function of the nucleus (Fisch, 1955; Hall, 1964) is at variance with available structural and functional information. The ventral cochlear nucleus does not exhibit zonal vulnerability to all pathogenic factors alike. For example, in the presence of systemic infectious intoxication, nerve cells may be affected throughout the brain generally and throughout the cochlear nuclei without topistic pattern.

Sequence of Degeneration of Components of the Cochlear Duct

Cochlear and VIIIth nerve disorders rarely if ever occur entirely separately or in pure form; it is difficult to define causal relationships and to identify a single structure as being responsible for a hearing disorder. It will be found in most cases, however, that the sensory cells are the dominant target in the earlier phases of a pathologic process involving the cochlea; severe hair cell injury tends in time to be followed by nerve degeneration (Johnsson, 1974). The rapidity and severity of the latter is affected somewhat by the state of preservation of supporting elements. The peripheral nerve fibers are found within folds of supporting cells, and the latter appear to exert a form of nutritive or protective influence.

Loudness Recruitment

The auditory test profiles of lesions affecting the cochlea, cochlear nerve, brain stem and temporal lobe have been presented (Liden, 1969). One of the features of concern is loudness recruitment. The latter is the accompaniment of an increase in intensity of sound by a disproportionate increase in the sensation of loudness (Mawson, 1963). This phenomenon has been considered in the past to result only from a lesion of the peripheral hearing organ (Dix, 1965; Hallpike, 1967). The previously-reviewed suggestion that the outer hair cells may, as a separate system, exercise a form of control over the inner hair cells (Spoendlin, 1972) could point to outer hair cell injury as a basis for the development of loudness recruitment. The appearance of recruitment in association with central lesions has, however, been reported (Carhart, 1967a,b; Dix and Hood, 1973; Liden, 1969) ; reference has been made to central recruitment (Liden, 1969). Most neural disorders exhibit some degree of recruitment (Priede and Coles, 1974). An explanation of this phenomenon has been offered on the basis of a dual audiologic system embracing the volley-place theory, with the volley mechanism accounting for lower frequencies while the place mechanism serves higher frequencies (Carhart, 1967a,b). High-tone hearing loss could then result from injury of the anatomic system serving higher frequencies. A structural alternative to the just-mentioned explanation is in relation to the participation of the octopoid cells of the inferior ventral cochlear nucleus in the inhibitory reflex circuit whose effector unit is the olivocochlear bundle (Osen, 1969a). If injury of the cochlear nucleus includes that of the octopoid cells, it is suggested that, the inhibitory mechanisms of concern being lost, central recruitment could develop (Hall, discussion on Dix and Hood, 1973).

Site of Involvement in Sensorineural Hearing Loss Caused by a Demyelinating Process

It has been pointed out that unilateral hearing loss in multiple sclerosis should result from demyelinating involvement of the central or glial portion of the cochlear nerve (Dix, 1965; Hallpike, 1967). A general principle of anatomy in relation to pathology is,

involved. An alternate possibility which must not be overlooked is that the cochlear nucleus and or trapezoid body may be included in a region of injury, thus effectively interrupting the afferent auditory pathway before fibers have crossed.

Transsynaptic Cell Degeneration

Transsynaptic cell injury has been described in the auditory pathway (Powell and Erulkar, 1962). The mechanism is not clear. Following unilateral experimental destruction of the ventral cochlear nucleus, neurons of the dorsal olivary complex may degenerate. The cells are reduced in size but apparently not in numbers. The cells of the medial dorsal olive do not share in the process, possibly because they receive bilateral nerve supply.

Variation in Normal Cell Population—Effect on Pathologic Appraisal

In persons with apparently normal hearing, foci may be encountered in which especially outer hair cells may be absent without apparent effect. Considerable variation between the two sides may be found in density and total numbers of sensory as well as spiral ganglion cells. The spiral ganglion may contain as many as 40 percent more or fewer cells than the average of nine other cases (Guild, 1932). The reserve capacity of the auditory pathway is to be reckoned with. It has been estimated that a residue of 20 to 25 percent of spiral ganglion neurons may be enough to provide pure tone sensitivity (Bredberg, 1968; Schuknecht and Woellner, 1955). The loss of nerve cells or fibers is felt earlier as one passes centrally. For example, in acoustic neurofibromas, speech discrimination may be impaired earlier than pure tone perception; more nerve cells or fibers are needed to serve the more complex, centrally-effected processes.

These foregoing features require that the attributing of hearing loss to the status observed within the auditory pathway in a single case be weighed judiciously. Counts of neurons, while potentially of statistical value in a sufficiently large series, are in particular, of questionable significance in single cases.

Effects of Interruption of Blood Supply

Vascular accidents in the labyrinth may account for sudden loss of function as in the central nervous system.

Experimental venous obstruction (Perlman and Kimura, 1957) leads to loss of hair cells, especially of the outer, inner hair cells being more resistant. The basal turn is most severely involved. Spiral ganglion cells are reduced, although less severely. The stria vascularis is especially susceptible and may be the first structure to show signs of injury. Dilatation of strial capillaries and edema of the epithelium occur promptly. Hemorrhages may develop within the epithelium and may extend into the scala media. The content of the endolymphatic sac may stain deeply.

Arterial occlusion (Perlman and Kimura, 1957) in general produces more rapid and profound changes. The entire end-organ degenerates as do also the spiral ganglion cells and the stria vascularis. The organ of Corti undergoes a process of shrinkage that may end in disappearance. A difficulty arises in that the appearance of the degenerated tissue is not unlike that encountered in human material altered by postmortem autolysis (Fernandez, 1958). This makes it difficult if not impossible to evaluate properly in the postmortem state the adequacy of the labyrinthine vascular system. Only the most advanced lesions would be reliably meaningful. The deleterious effects of arterial occlusion produced by injection of a suspension of barium sulfate can be inhibited with administration of vasodilating agents (Suga, Preston and Snow, 1970).

Autolysis and Artifact

More so in the cochlea than in the brain, the ever present danger of the occurrence of postmortem autolysis and of the production of artifact requires the careful exclusion of such changes before accepting histologic alterations as being truly pathologic. As few as half of processed inner ears may be well enough preserved to be satisfactory for study.

Postmortem change may be seen in the organ of Corti as a feathery type of dissolution. Another variant is a form of shrinkage or inspissation (Fernandez, 1958). Artifacts may resemble the features of pathologic states or vice versa; this has been observed in vascular occlusion as just mentioned. Such alterations tend to affect tissues similarly throughout the cochlea. It is in support of the presence of a truly pathologic state if a selectively regional or zonal distribution is observed.

Pyknosis may represent artifact rather than true abnormality. This alteration is seen in the form of dark cells (no relation to electron-dense material). It may result from the handling of un-fixed tissues at postmortem, resulting in disruption, thereby per-mitting shrinkage (Cammermeyer, 1960). This will occur less often if fixation by injection has been performed, i.e. embalming, especially if the examination is delayed for as much as four hours to permit fixation to occur; otherwise the injection will have cor-respondingly less effect. In experimental work, prompt fixation by intravital perfusion has been found essential to avoidance of the very early occurrence, otherwise, of autolytic changes (Jordan, Pinheiro, Chiba and Jimenez, 1973).

Labyrinthine Ossification

As a sequel to inflammation within the labyrinth or following injury, the cavities may ossify owing to a tendency of the endosteal layer to overreact under such circumstances. The process may oc-clude the inner ear completely (Altmann, 1965; Sugiura and Pa-parella, 1967).

Deafness of Sudden Onset

Sudden hearing loss (Schuknecht, Benitez, Beekhuis, Igarashi and Singleton, 1962; Snow, 1973) is so classified if it occurs over the course of as long as some hours or a few days. The cause may not always be apparent, but in most instances etiology is accounted for under the various categories which include infection (espe-cially viral), trauma (including factors of force and of excessive sound level) and vascular accident.

Acupuncture and Hearing

Some success has been reported with the treatment of sensor-ineural deafness with acupuncture (Kao, Baker, Leung, Slippen, Ampolsakdi and Lapidot, 1973; Peng, 1974). Contrary results have been obtained (Fairbanks, Wallenberg and Webb, 1974; Marcus and Goldenberg, 1974; Rintlemann, Oyer, Forbord and Flowers, 1974).

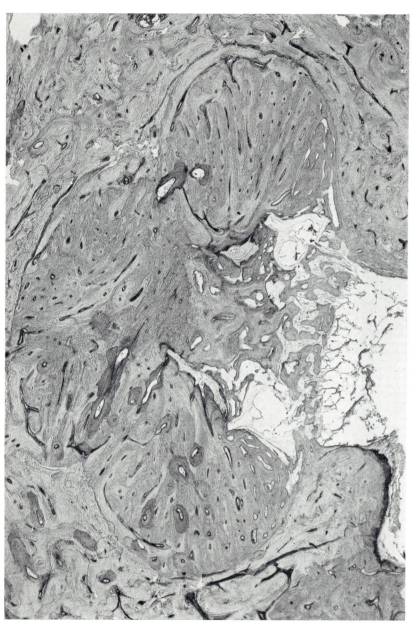

Figure 38. Labyrinthine ossification. New bone formation has obliterated the scalae. This occurred following a febrile illness thought to be meningitis, apparently with accompanying labyrinthitis, following which the patient was profoundly deaf. Illustration courtesy Schuknecht, *Pathology of the Ear*, Harvard University Press, 1974.

Chapter 4 _____

DEVELOPMENTAL ABNORMALITIES— CONGENITAL AND GENETIC DISORDERS

C ONGENITAL, GENETIC and hereditary factors may be combined in the production of hearing loss, and their respective participation may not always be separable. Complexity is the rule rather than the exception. As many as ninety hereditary categories have been recognized (Konigsmark, 1969), and the list is extended periodically (Shambaugh, 1967b). In the present discussion some of the more salient features are presented.

Pathologic lesions resulting in deafness may be produced by failures of the structure(s) of concern to develop, interruption of development, or injury to tissue(s) already developed.

PATHOLOGIC TYPES OF MALDEVELOPMENT

The resulting states of pathologic involvement as affecting the inner ear (Lindsay, 1973a) are grouped in four main categories. These have been designated by workers' names, an unsatisfactory procedure for reasons including the one that such names are applied to what in essence appear to be stages of a process. The principle of numerical staging is suggested here, with inclusion of names (Beal, Davey and Lindsay, 1967; Igarashi, 1972) for the sake of traditional orientation.

Type I (Michel); Lack of development of the inner ear.

Type II (Mondini-Alexander): Development of only a single tube or a flattened and shortened cochlea with bony architectural abnormalities and enlarged saccule and endolymphatic system.

Type III (Bing-Siebenmann): Normal bony labyrinth, but

anomalous labyrinthine sensory epithelium and/or membranous labyrinth.

Type IV (Scheibe): Normal bony labyrinth; degeneration of pars inferior (cochleosaccular degeneration) of the membranous labyrinth. About 70 percent of cases of congenital abnormality are of this type (Igarashi, 1972).

In addition, categories are recognized relative to accompanying malformations of parts other than the inner ear (Igarashi, 1972; Konigsmark, 1970).

Type V (Siebenmann): With malformations of middle ear and external ear canal.

Type VI: With microtia and atresia of external meatus.

The relation of embryogenesis to the type of lesion is important with regard especially to the development of the different parts of the labyrinth according to certain timetables, phylogenetic as well as embryologic.

In the effort to determine etiology in a given case of deafness (Paparella and Capps, 1973) one should endeavor to establish whether the hearing loss is congenital or acquired after birth. In general, congenital deafness implies aplasia or dysgenesis of the organ of Corti and related structures. In such cases the deafness should not be progressive. Hearing loss of delayed onset relates to degenerative changes of the sensory organ and may be progressive. The genetic versus nongenetic character of the disorder should also be established where possible; this may be difficult. As was indicated, the presence of accompanying anomalies is also of concern.

One of the main difficulties encountered in the study of cases of the type(s) presently under discussion is the all too frequent lack of an accurate history and audiometric data.

CONGENITAL MALDEVELOPMENTS OF GESTATIONAL ORIGIN

In comparatively recent years, the relation of certain detectable pathogenic factors to congenital hearing loss has been shown, permitting the removal of some cases from the sizeable idiopathic reservoir.

Rubella (German Measles)

Congenital deafness resulting from maternal rubella (Carruthers, 1945; Paparella and Capps, 1973; Ward, Honrubia and Moore, 1968; Wolf and Cowen, 1972) has been encountered in epidemics. In some cases the maternal infection was not known, the diagnosis being made serologically (Karmody, 1969). The introduction of immune prophylaxis has resulted in decrease of case frequency, with commensurate unreliability of current estimates of incidence. Reported loss of hearing ranges from 2 to 70 percent in cases of known maternal rubella. This depends somewhat on stage of embryonic development at the time of infection. In the presence of infection during the first trimester of gestation there is a high probability of some degree of hearing loss. In cases of infection before the end of the sixth week of pregnancy, damage to the fetus is likely to be widespread and may involve eyes (microphthalmia, cataract, glaucoma, retinopathy), cardiovascular system (ventricular septal defect, patent ductus arteriosus) and brain (microcephaly, mental retardation). There may be stunting of growth. At the end of six weeks these organ systems may escape; even slightly later the cochlear duct and saccule may be affected while the utricle and semicircular ducts, structures that develop earlier, may be unaltered. The organ of Corti may fail to develop, and the tectorial membrane may be rolled up and ensheathed and may be found in the inner sulcus or on the spiral limbus or broadly adherent to a flattened organ of Corti. The stria vascularis may be relatively shallow and avascular. The vestibular membrane may be collapsed; tectorial and vestibular membranes may be missing entirely. The spiral ganglion and cochlear nerve tend to be comparatively intact.

After the conclusion of the third month of gestation the fetus may escape injury; however, cases are reported of involvement of the cochlear duct in maternal rubella wherein the process appears to be one of injury to tissues which are well-formed, suggesting a later or continuing state of infection of the fetal cochlea, the histopathologic pattern resembling that of postnatal viral infection (Lindsay, Carruthers, Hemenway and Harrison, 1953; Ward, Honrubia and Moore, 1968). Aside from outright severe brain

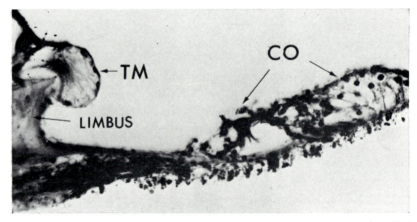

Figure 39. Prenatal maternal rubella. The tectorial membrane (TM) is rolled up, covered by a single layer of cells, and retracted to the lip of the degenerated limbus. Corti's organ (CO) had been fairly well developed. Illustration courtesy Lindsay, *Ann Otol, 82*:Suppl. 5, 1973.

destruction from encephalitis (Wolf and Cowen, 1972), central auditory imperception may be encountered; this may be the only apparent manifestation of the disorder (Ames, Plotkin, Winchester and Atkins, 1970).

Deafness in congenital rubella tends to be attended by a flat audiometric pattern said to reflect general arrest of development of the hearing organ (Fisch, 1955, Miller, Rabinowitz and Cohen, 1971).

Encephalitis of congenital origin may be produced by a number of infectious agents. This occurs notably in cytomegalic viral disease (Davis, 1969; Myers and Stool, 1968) and toxoplasmosis (Keleman, 1958; Wolf and Cowen, 1972), although not often resulting in hearing loss which is not obscured by involvement of the brain as a whole.

Kernicterus

The term *kernicterus* will be employed for the disorder now to be discussed, although with the disadvantage of inconstancy, certain cases showing no pigmentation of the cerebral tissues. Consequent to the use of immune globulin, exchange transfusion and ultraviolet irradiation, kernicterus has become increasingly rare. When it is encountered in a fatal case the tissues, however, stand as the valuable product of an experiment of nature and provide an unusual opportunity for the study of pathogenic principles of concern.

Kernicterus is encountered notably as a sequel to erythroblastosis fetalis resulting from immune reaction of maternal antibodies to fetal erythrocytes, most often D-positive, the mother being D-negative; the reaction leads to hemolysis. The disorder is accordingly genetic and hereditary; indeed, it could be discussed under a number of headings.

The basic pathogenic factor in kernicterus is anoxia (Buch, Tygstrup and Jørgensen, 1966; Dublin, 1949; Meriwether, Hager and Scholz, 1955). If it is not the sole factor, the anoxia predisposes the tissues to any further injury which may be caused by bile pigment (Chen, Wang, Tsan and Chen, 1966); degenerated tissues tend to be impregnated by the pigment. The toxic action of bilirubin appears to include the uncoupling of oxidative phosphorylation in mitochondria (Ernster, Herlin and Zetterström, 1957). The level of total serum bilirubin appears not to be as important as that of the unconjugated portion. This is influenced, among other factors, by the ability of the liver to conjugate the pigment through the use of glucuronyl transferase, whose low level in the livers of premature infants tends to expose these subjects to the effect of bilirubin (Blanc and Johnson, 1959; Day, 1961; Johnson, Garcia, Figueroa and Sarmiento, 1961). Kernicterus may develop apart from erythroblastosis (Aidin, Corner and Tovey, 1950; Crigler and Najjar, 1952; Forster and McCormack, 1944), usually in association with prematurity (Gerrard, 1952; Gooch, 1961).

In children who survive erythroblastosis, the serious residuals are principally neuropsychiatric; they may include mental retardation, emotional instability, muscular spasticity of extrapyramidal type, choreoathetosis and convulsions (Dublin, 1951). Sensorineural hearing loss may occur (Byers, Paine and Crothers, 1955; Cavanaugh, 1954); estimates of percentile incidence are quite variable, ranging from 80 percent (Crabtree and Gerrard, 1950) to minimal, some contributors finding the disorder to be interpretive more than perceptive (Cohen, 1956). The fact is that the central portion of the auditory pathway may be involved at all levels (Dublin, 1951).

The hearing loss tends to be of high-tone type (Cavanaugh, 1954; Crabtree and Gerrard, 1950); the audiometric curve varies, but tends to be downward-sloping, indicating a selective injury of tissue previously formed (Fisch, 1955). A characteristic mean audiometric curve shows maximal loss at 2000 to 4000 cps (Matkin and Carhart, 1966). The pathologic study of tissues from post-kernicteric subjects with hearing loss documented with audiogram has not yet been reported.

At postmortem the brains of kernicteric newborns show grossly golden pigmentation of those centers especially affected by anoxia: notably the lenticular and dentate nuclei and hippocampus (Dublin, 1949). The subthalamic nuclei also tend to be involved (Meriwether, Hager and Scholz, 1955). Various medullary nuclei may be outlined; this may include the cochlear nuclei, but the vestibular group is affected more notably.

The anoxic topistic distribution is maintained microscopically also. In addition to the aforementioned structures, the cerebral cortex may be involved together, variably, with adjoining white matter. The basis for the anoxic distribution is not understood. The affected nerve cell bodies show varying stages and types of injury, ranging to disappearance. They, together with portions of the intervening neuropil, may show, in favorable cases, deposit of pigment, the latter having survived the action of solvents and reagents incident to histotechnical processing (*see* Figures 40 A, B, & C).

On review of the structures of the auditory pathway, the cochlear elements show no regularly and clearly detectable alteration (Dublin, 1974; Buch, Tygstrup and Jørgensen, 1966; Gerrard, 1952). The central portion of the pathway is involved, not outstandingly, but in keeping with the degree of alteration found throughout the brain generally (Buch, Tygstrup and Jørgensen, 1966) (*see* Figure 41).

The cochlear nuclear complex is affected variably in degree but characteristically as to pattern of distribution (Dublin, 1974). The dorsal cochlear nucleus is essentially unaltered. The most impressive nerve cell injury is observed in the ventral cochlear nucleus, especially the superior ventral division. If the alteration is severe, the entire superior ventral nucleus may be injured; in such cases there will be total deafness. If the process is moderate in severity so that the nucleus is only partly effaced, cell injury will be found in a zone within the dorsal portion of the superior ventral nucleus, although sparing the dorsalmost portion. This zone corresponds strikingly with the 2000 to 4000 cps segment of the audiogram if the latter is oriented in relation to the superior ventral cochlear nucleus so that low frequencies correspond to ventral and high frequencies correspond to dorsal. Findings of this type are in keeping with the existence of a low frequency-ventral to high frequency-dorsal tonotopic pattern in the ventral cochlear nucleus. This nucleus, further, appears to share with the cochlea the feature of a zonal susceptibility to injury of that portion serving higher frequencies (Dublin, 1974). The pathogenic mechanism for this is not understood (*see* Figures 42 A & B).

The spheroid cells appear chiefly affected; they appear relatively susceptible to injury. Variable stages of degeneration are seen with formation of empty spaces where the related cells have disappeared. Injury of spheroid cells appears to be the basis of sensorineural hearing loss of central or so-called nuclear type. The other cell types also are involved, but less strikingly. Multipolar cells tend to become pyknotic, a form of alteration to be regarded with interpretive reservation. The fibers of the trapezoid body appear reduced consequent to injury of the cells of origin of the fibers in the ventral cochlear nucleus.

The dorsal olivary nuclear complex, inferior colliculi, medial geniculate bodies and auditory cortex appear altered variably, serving as a basis, increasing with passage centrally, for the associational or interpretive features of the hearing loss.

Nerve cell alteration of the just-mentioned active or acute type is more amenable to evaluation than is the status in the late posterythroblastotic state, in which the less reliable feature of diminished numbers of nerve cells must be evaluated together with the presence of gliosis. Specific auditory pathway studies of such tissues have not as yet been reported.

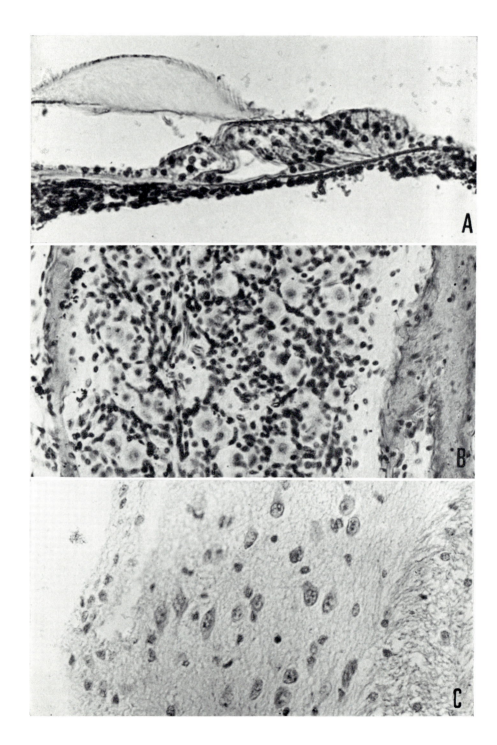

Loudness recruitment, traditionally considered a feature of injury of the peripheral hearing organ, is characteristically present in kernicterus in which, as has been shown, the sensorineural lesion is in the ventral cochlear nucleus. In order to explain this finding the volley-place theory is adduced, suggesting that two hearing mechanisms exist, one (volley-sensitive) for low tones (from 300 cps downward), and one (place-sensitive) for higher tones (from 1300 cps upward), with a zone of transition in between (Carhart, 1967a,b). It is pointed out that in the mean characteristic audiogram in kernicterus there is a plateau of relatively good hearing for low frequencies, with transition across one of the octaves between 250 and 2000 cps to a plateau of relatively poor acuity for higher frequencies. Loudness recruitment, however, has been reported in the presence of brain stem lesions (Dix and Hood, 1973); a form of central recruitment has been recognized (Liden, 1969). This could be explained by the inclusion of the octopoid cells among those injured in the ventral cochlear nucleus (Hall, discussion on Dix and Hood, 1973).

Effects of Maternal Ingestion of Thalidomide

The fetal teratogenic effects of maternal ingestion of thalidomide may include deformities affecting the inner ear (Schuknecht, 1974 (*see* Figures 43 A & B).

Arnold-Chiari Deformity

In meningocele associated with spina bifida, in flat base, or without apparent cause, the medulla may be found within the foramen magnum, and its ventral surface may be compressed. The acoustic nerve may be bent over the margin of the internal acoustic meatus or may be compressed or stretched. The cochlear nuclei may be compressed. Auditory symptoms may appear in as many as 20 percent of cases (Rydell and Pulec, 1971) (*see* Figures 44 A & B).

Figure 40. Two-day-old erythroblastotic infant.
Figure 40A. Slightly tangential section of organ of Corti.
Figure 40B. Spiral ganglion.
Figure 40C. Fusiform cells of dorsal cochlear nucleus.
These tissues are essentially unaltered.

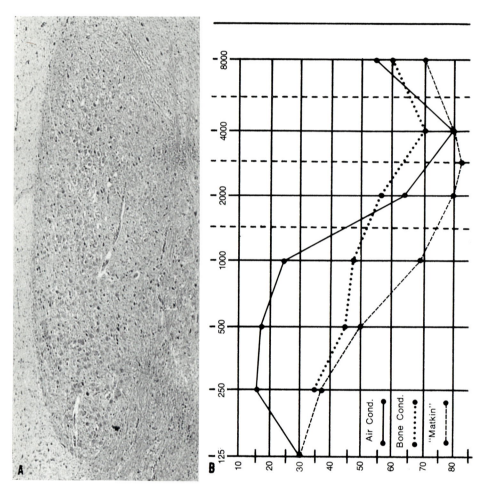

Figure 41. Same case as in Figure 40.

Figure 41A. Transverse section through the superior ventral cochlear nucleus. Figure 41B. A characteristic audiogram in post-erythroblastosis hearing loss (Crabtree and Gerrard, 1950) and the Matkin audiogram (Matkin and Carhart, 1966), representing the mean of twenty-two such cases, are turned to a vertical position for comparison with Figure 41A.

Even at the provided magnification, cellular injury is seen that corresponds in distribution to the downward deflection of the audiometric tracing. Illustration from Dublin, *Arch Otolaryngol, 100:* 355, 1974, copyright American Medical Association.

CONGENITAL GENETIC DEAFNESS

Some forms of genetically-determined sensorineural hearing loss are not necessarily hereditary but result from chromosomal nondisjunction during meiosis in gamete formation, resulting in an extra chromosome within a pair, or trisomy. Recognized autosomal trisomy syndromes designated by the numbered chomosomal pairs subject to involvement include 13-15 (D-trisomy), 17-18 (E-trisomy) and 21-22 (mongolism or Down's syndrome). The syndromes exhibit characteristic anomalous patterns; the considerable numbers of expected abnormalities have been listed (Kos, Schuknecht and Singer, 1966; Maniglia, Wolff and Herques, 1970; Sando, Bergstrom, Wood and Hemenway, 1970). Reports of pathologic studies are few. In two infants with 13-15 trisomy there was no response to sound. Type IV (cochleosaccular, Scheibe) anomaly was found. The organ of Corti was defective or missing. The tectorial membrane was displaced. The vestibular membrane was depressed or missing. The stria vascularis was atrophic or cystic. Severity of these alterations was greater toward the base. Defective formation of the modiolus was less notable; the spiral ganglion appeared well-formed throughout (Kos, Schuknecht and Singer, 1966). In one case there was the added finding of a teratomatous growth within the internal auditory canal composed of striated muscle and nerve fibers (Maniglia, Wolff and Herques, 1970).

In 18 trisomy, defective formation of the modiolus appeared to be more appreciable, with deficient spiral ganglion (Kos, Schuknecht and Singer, 1966). In one case outer hair cells were also found missing toward the base (Sando, Bergstrom, Wood and Hemenway, 1970).

Anomalous formation of the central pathway reported in trisomy included heterotopic foci of neurons and undifferentiated glial cells in the ventral cochlear nucleus (Terplan, Sandberg and Aceto, 1966).

HEREDITARY DEAFNESS

General Features

Approximately 50 percent of deafness appears to be hereditary, and in the majority of cases, recessive. Such a disorder in most in-

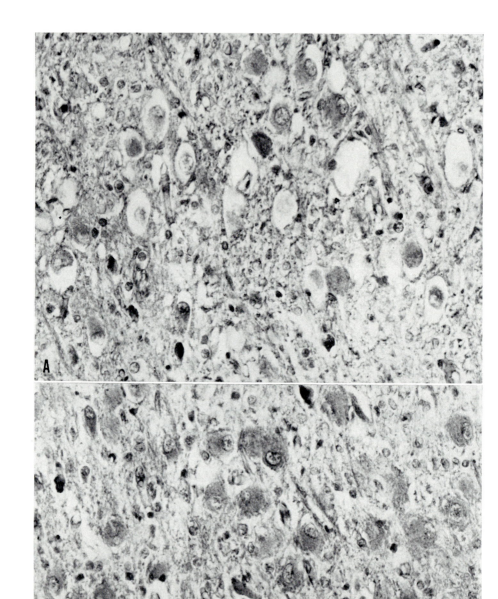

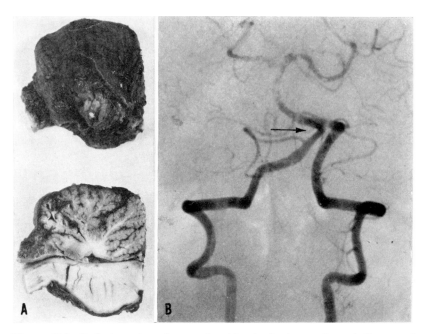

Figure 43A. Left lateral surface and midsagittal views of cerebellum and brain stem in Arnold-Chiari deformity. Cerebellar coning and compression of the ventral surface of the medulla are observed. Cochlear nerves and nuclei are included among the structures injured in such cases. Illustration from Dublin, *Fundamentals of Neuropatholgy*, Ed. II, Charles C Thomas, 1967.

Figure 43B. Vertebral arteriogram showing lateral displacement of vertebral arteries (arrow), one of them lying in the cerebellopontine recess between nerves VII and VIII with symptoms of cerebellopontine recess involvement. Roentgenogram courtesy Dr. Thomas H. Newton.

Figure 42. Same case as in Figures 40 and 41. High power views of upper and lower fields of the superior ventral cochlear nucleus. In Figure 42B there is some expected edema, but the spheroid cells are essentially well preserved. In Figure 42A, its maximal degree corresponding to about 3,000 cps in the audiogram, there is notable tissue injury showing various stages of degeneration, especially of the spheroid cells. Illustration from Dublin, *Arch Otolaryngol, 100:* 355, 1974, copyright American Medical Association.

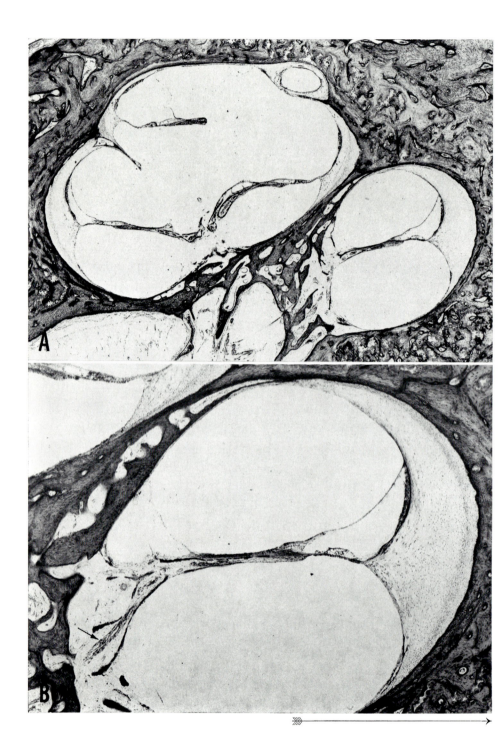

stances is not amenable to treatment. Roughly one third of heredi-tary deafness is associated with recognized syndromes (Paparella and Capps, 1973).

Inherited deafness is classified further as being congenital versus delayed in onset, and as occurring alone or with other abnormalities. Cases that are of neonatal onset are divided into the previously presented structural types (traditionally, Michel, Mondini, Bing-Siebenmann, and Scheibe [Lindsay, 1973a; Paparella and Capps, 1973]). The resultant pathologic status in each category is some-what the same as that encountered in trisomy syndrome. The basis of subclassification is, as was indicated previously, essentially that of stages or degrees of involvement of a process. Less severe deficiency of formation of the structures of the cochlear duct will accordingly be found in type IV cases (Scheibe), offering greater likelihood of benefit from acoustic amplification, since there may be some degree of formation of the cochlear duct with resultant capacity for hear-ing in the low frequencies (Paparella and Capps, 1973).

Deafness of neonatal onset accompanying disorders of other systems offers a basis for the recognition of potentially numerous syndromes (Konigsmark, 1969, 1970). They include Waarden-burg's disease, albinism, hyperpigmentation, onychodystrophy and the syndromes of Jervell and Usher (Paparella and Capps, 1973).

Pendred's Syndrome

Pendred's syndrome (nonendemic goiter) (Illum, Kiaer, Hvid-berg-Hansen and Søndergaard, 1972; Paparella and Capps, 1973) appears to deserve separate recognition. It accounts for as many as 10 percent of cases of recessive deafness. The patient usually is deaf at birth; the thyroid enlargement which characteristically appears becomes evident more often during adolescence. Normally the ad-

Figure 44. Trisomy 18 abnormality.
Figure 44A. Partition between middle and apical turns missing with forma-tion of scala communis. Spiral ganglion also missing.
Figure 44B. Total absence of spiral ganglion cells and afferent nerve fibers. Small bundle of nerve fibers (arrow) probably efferent.

Illustrations courtesy Schuknecht (Kos, Schuknecht and Singer), *Arch Otolaryngol, 83:*439, 1966, copyright American Medical Association.

ministration of perchlorate induces the release of inorganic-bound iodine from the thyroid. In Pendred's syndrome there is a fall in this activity. It is presumed to result from a defect in the peroxidase system (Illum, Kiaer, Hvidberg-Hansen and Søndergaard, 1972). The inner ear shows type II abnormality (Mondini); only the basal turn is developed, the remainder forming a common cavity. There is considered to be a fault during the seventh week in the development of the modiolus. There is a discrepancy in relation to the accepted tonotopicity of the cochlea since the deafness is high-frequency (Illum, Kiaer, Hvidberg-Hansen and Søndergaard, 1972).

Usher's Syndrome

Sensorineural deafness may occur in association with retinitis pigmentosa (Schuknecht, 1974).

Hereditary Deafness of Late Onset

Those hereditary disorders which become manifest after birth represent the deterioration of a preformed organ of Corti and usually are progressive.

Familial Progressive Sensorineural Deafness

This disorder (Paparella and Capps, 1973) constitutes essentially the category of hereditary deafness of late onset unaccompanied by lesions of other systems. It is familial in incidence. The audiometric pattern may show high-tone, flat or basin-shaped loss. The deafness usually is bilateral and is considered to be autosomal dominant. Onset is in childhood, adolescence or early adulthood; the disorder progresses in severity during adulthood. Histologic studies have shown deficiencies of the basal turn of the cochlea affecting the organ of Corti, spiral ganglion and stria vascularis (Paparella and Capps, 1973).

Hereditary Deafness of Late Onset Associated With Other Abnormalities

The number of recognized members of this general category is potentially large (Konigsmark, 1969, 1970). A few will be discussed here.

ALPORT'S SYNDROME. This multisystem disorder (Alport, 1927; Fujita and Hayden, 1969; Miller, Joseph, Cozad and McCabe, 1970; Myers and Tyler, 1972; Paparella and Capps, 1973) is hereditary (dominant) and familial. Bilaterally symmetrical, high-tone sensorineural hearing loss is accompanied by glomerulonephritis. Onset is frequently in preadolescence and may exhibit slowly progressive deafness before the recognition of the renal disorder. The audiometric curve tends to be gently declining. Males are affected more frequently and severely and seldom live beyond the age of thirty. Females exhibit deafness, that may be relatively mild, and hematuria; they tend to live to old age.

There is a lack of consistent pathologic inner ear alterations. Some reports indicate no recognized change. Others indicate some degree of degeneration of the organ of Corti and stria vascularis, especially in the basal turn. More work is needed. Particularly lacking are well-controlled central auditory studies. Lipid-laden cells are found in the renal cortex.

KLIPPEL-FEIL SYNDROME. This autosomal hereditary disorder (Palant and Carter, 1972) is more often dominant, less often recessive. It is manifested as a triad of limitation of movement of the head, short neck and low posterior hair line, often associated with other congenital anomalies. There are skeletal defects that may include fusion of upper cervical vertebrae with one another and with the occiput. Other anomalies may be encountered, including spina bifida and meningocele. Profound sensorineural deafness may occur in as many as 30 percent of cases secondary to abnormal inner ear development. This may involve the bony as well as the membranous labyrinth and the auditory nerve (McLay and Maran, 1969).

MISCELLANEOUS SYNDROMES. Other syndromes in which sensorineural deafness may occur (Paparella and Capps, 1973) include Hurler's syndrome *(gargoylism)*, Refsum's disease and Alstrom's disease (retinitis pigmentosa appears in the two latter categories). Von Recklinghausen's disease is encountered in some cases of acoustic neurofibroma. The osseous involvement in Paget's disease, inherited as an autosomal dominant, results primarily in conductive deafness; the compact cochlear bone tends to be resistive. In some cases involvement of the cochlea produces degeneration of the organ of Corti and stria vascularis. The audiogram may show a high frequency drop or a relatively flat pattern (Clemis, Boyles, Harford and Petasnick, 1967; Paparella and Capps, 1973) .

Chapter 5 _____

INFECTIONS — INFECTIOUS INTOXICATIONS — IMMUNE DISORDERS

THE STRUCTURES of the auditory pathway share, along with other tissues of the body, in the general involvement of systemic infections, and the listing of all such processes would entail a recapitulation of a segment of general pathology. In the discussion to follow some of the more salient features will be presented, together with special discussion of processes that affect the auditory pathway in such a way as to produce clinically appreciable deafness. Undoubtedly there are many cases in which hearing loss occurs but is overshadowed by the generally incapacitating nature of the disorder.

A clinical diagnosis of labyrinthitis frequently is made in the presence of symptoms of uncertain etiology. There is particular need for well-controlled auditory pathway studies that include the central nervous system to provide better understanding of toxic-infective and related processes that lead to disordered hearing directly or indirectly.

SEROUS LABYRINTHITIS—MENINGISMUS— TOXIC ENCEPHALITIS AND NEURITIS

Serous labyrinthitis, a nonpurulent inflammation of the inner ear, appears to represent a stage of diffusion of infectious toxin, possibly as an antecedent to actual invasion by bacteria (Paparella and Capps, 1973). The disorder tends to be transient, and human tissues are not often available for pathologic study. Hearing may be impaired, but not markedly so; severe loss of hearing indicates the

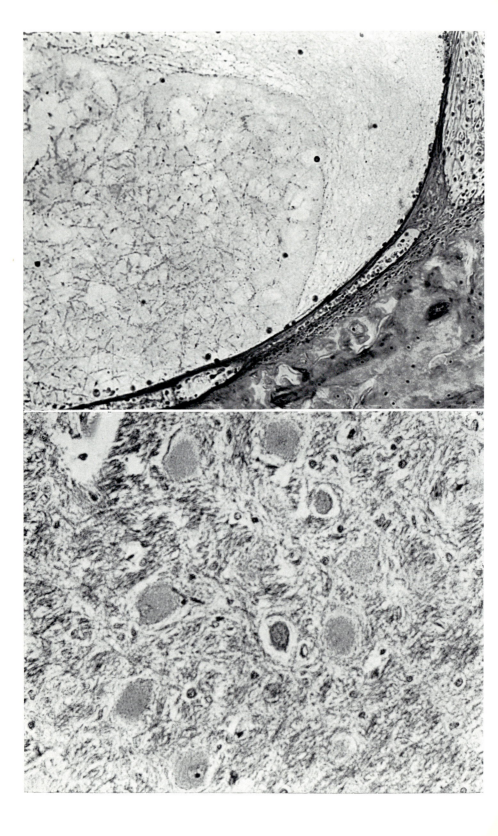

liability of appearance of suppuration. The relative normalcy of hearing is in keeping with absence of notable alteration of endolymph, while perilymph is visably involved; an eosinophilic precipiate appears in the form of serofibrinous strands resulting from elevation of protein.

Especially in children, increased production of cerebrospinal fluid in the presence of high fever is manifested clinically as meningismus, symptomatic equivalent of meningitis without inflammation per se.

Toxic encephalitis and neuritis are attended by the complicating influence of infective vascular lesions and factors of metabolic imbalance. Virtually any systemic infection may serve as cause. The main gross features are edema and congestion of the cerebral tissues, with variable hemorrhages, from petechial to massive.

Specific histologic studies of auditory pathway tissues are needed. The neural portions of these tissues, including the spiral ganglion and cochlear nerve, doubtless are affected like those of the remainder of the brain. In general, in addition to congestion and edema, nerve cells show changes of moderate and usually reversible degree such as cloudy swelling or mild vacuolation. Cell loss is slight or inconstant. Swelling and proliferation of oligodendrocytes tends to occur. There is noteworthy involvement of blood vessels; in active stages there is swelling and proliferation of endothelium, particularly of capillaries and small arterioles. Vessel walls may become necrotic, and hemorrhages, large and small, may occur. The auditory nerve may share in general neuroradiculoneuritis; pathologic studies are needed.

In the foregoing process there appears to be no zonal predilection of involvement of the cochlear nucleus.

Figure 45 (upper). Serous labyrinthitis, scala tympani (cat). A fibrillar precipitate is seen. Illustration courtesy Paparella and Capps in Paparella and Shumwick (Eds.): *Otolaryngolgoy,* W.B. Saunders, 1973.

Figure 45 (lower). Reaction of spheroid cells, superior ventral cochlear nucleus, to infectious toxin of pneumonia. Cytoplasm is swollen and homogenous; nuclei are eccentric. Intercellular tissue is edematous. The effect was observed evenly throughout the nucleus without zonal selection.

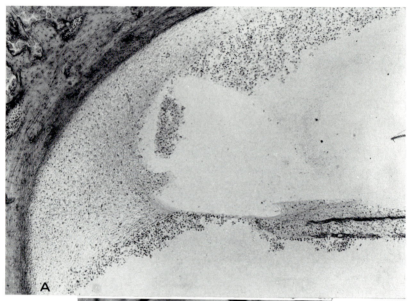

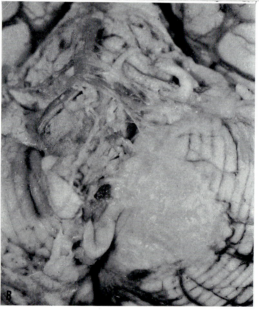

PURULENT LABYRINTHITIS AND MENINGITIS

Purulent labyrinthitis may involve any of the pyogenic bacteria including streptococcus, staphylococcus, meningococcus, pneumococcus, hemophilus, pseudomonas and proteus (Igarashi, 1972). The infection may enter the labyrinth by spread from (1) the tympanic cavity; entry may be by penetration of the windows (Paparella, Oda, Hiraide and Brady, 1972). It may result from erosion by cholesteatoma or tumor or from fracture. In penetrating injuries of the tympanic membrane the stapes may be driven into the vestibule. The causative injury may be iatrogenic. (2) meninges, in purulent meningitis (Igarashi, Saito, Alford, Filippone and Smith, 1974). Entry may be through the base of the modiolus or the cochlear aqueduct. Estimates of incidence of labyrinthitis in meningococcic meningitis is about 4 percent. This form of meningitis appears to be among the more common causes of profound deafness in children acquired after the end of the neonatal period; estimates of deafness in epidemic meningitis range from 4 to 37 percent (Paparella and Capps, 1973). (This would include cases of injury to cochlear nerve and/or nucleus and postinflammatory adhesions, etc.) (3) the blood stream, considered least common.

Purulent exudate is found in all parts of the labyrinth (Paparella and Sugiura, 1967). The sensory elements degenerate and disappear, followed by the supporting cells; the stria vascularis is effaced, and the vestibular membrane may collapse (Igarashi, 1972). If the patient does not succumb to cerebellar abscess or meningitis, healing occurs, the stages being attended by production of exudate, granulation tissue, fibrous tissue and bone, respectively

---

Figure 46A. Labyrinthitis complicating otitis media. Inflammatory exudate is seen especially in the scala vestibuli, and the organ of Corti and vestibular membrane have been destroyed.

Figure 46B. Purulent staphylococcic meningitis involving base of brain following fracture through the sphenoid sinus. In case of survival, meningeal adhesions could form with blockage of flow of cerebrospinal fluid in addition to residuals of destruction of tissue by the infectious process. Illustration from Dublin, *Fundamentals of Neuropathology*, Ed II, Charles C Thomas, 1967.

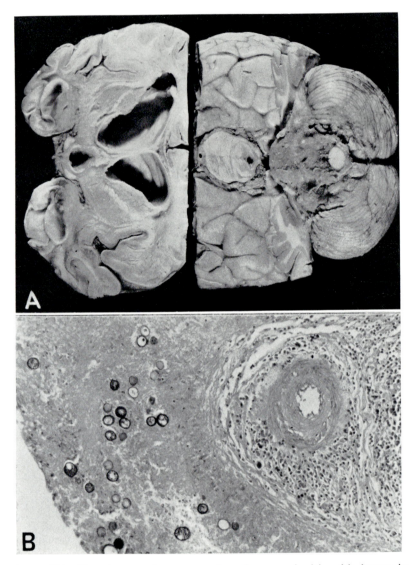

Figure 47A. Chronic granulomatous tuberculous meningitis with heavy involvement of the pontomedullary region including cochlear nerves and nuclei and with internal hydrocephalus. Illustration from Dublin, *Fundamentals of Neuropathology*, Ed. II, Charles C Thomas, 1967.

Figure 47B. Coccidioidal granuloma in cerebellopontine angle recess adjoining nerve VIII.

(Shambaugh, 1967a). The new bone formation may obliterate the labyrinth. It represents a trait of excessive reaction of the labyrinthine endosteum to injury.

Purulent labyrinthitis produces total deafness that tends to be permanent.

Purulent meningitis may be attended by cranial nerve involvement including cochlear. Especially following infection producing heavy exudate about the base of the brain, in cases of survival, adhesions may form; hydrocephalus may result.

INFECTIONS WITH MOLDS

In addition to variable lesions of the central portions of the auditory pathway the cochlear nerve may be involved in meningitis due to molds including cryptococcus or coccidioides. Specific auditory pathway studies are needed in this category as in so many others.

VIRAL INFECTIONS

Viral labyrinthitis (Strauss and Davis, 1973) appears to be one of the main causes of sudden deafness (Beal, Hemenway and Lindsay, 1967; Lindsay, 1959; Schuknecht, Benitez, Beekhuis *et al.*, 1962; Snow, 1973). Congenital rubella was discussed previously. The most common forms of acquired viral labyrinthitis are those of mumps, measles and influenza.

Deafness in mumps is among the commonest causes of acquired unilateral sensorineural deafness in children, accounting for 3 to 5 percent of deaf mutes (Lindsay, Davey and Ward, 1960). The structures of the cochlear duct appear severely damaged, especially toward the base. The organ of Corti appears degenerated. The tectorial membrane is particularly and characteristically deformed; it may appear rolled up into a displaced round (as seen in cross section) mass covered with a single layer of mesothelium, or may be flatly adherent to the injured organ of Corti. In severe cases the organ of Corti is missing entirely. The stria vascularis appears atrophic. The vestibular membrane may be collapsed. The neurons of the spiral ganglion are relatively preserved. Mumps meningoen-

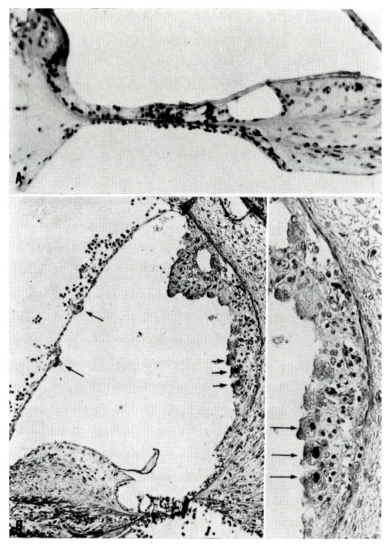

Figure 48A. Viral labryinthitis resulting in sudden deafness. Tectorial membrane is distorted and is adherent to the injured organ of Corti. Small visible portion of stria vacularis appears affected. Illustration courtesy Schuknecht (with Igarashi and Gacek), *Acta Otolaryngol, 59:*154, 1965.

Figure 48B. Cytomegalovirus infection of cochlear duct. Enlarged cells containing large, darkly-staining inclusions (arrows) are seen in stria vascularis and on under surface of vestibular membrane. After Davis, *Ann Otol, 78:* 1179, 1969.

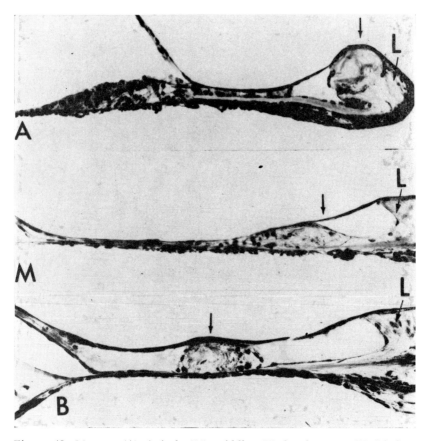

Figure 49. Mumps. (A) Apical, (M) middle, (B) basal turns. (L) Limbus. Vestibular membrane is depressed, obliterating scala media in middle and basal turns. Tectorial membrane is degenerated and is rolled into a ball. Organ of Corti is absent in middle and basal turns; in apical turn, cells are injured but can be partially identified. Illustration courtesy Lindsay (with Davey and Ward), *Ann Otol, 69*:918, 1960.

cephalitis entails a marked lymphocytic response. Recovery is the rule. Central nervous system auditory studies are few; any such involvement is overshadowed by that of the labyrinth.

Labyrinthitis in measles is less common than the foregoing. Bacterial infection may occur as a complication. The hearing impairment tends to be bilaterally symmetrical, high-tone. The path-

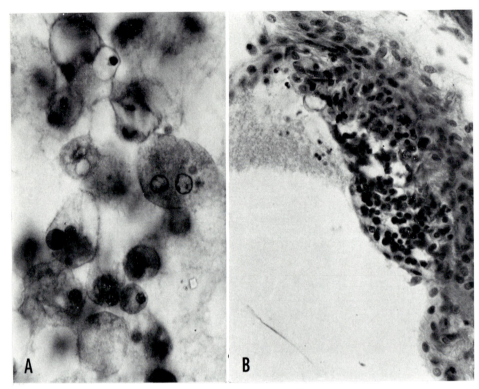

Figure 50. Measles. Figure 50A. Large multinucleated macrophages appear within labyrinth.
Figure 50B. Inflammation, with edema and cellular infiltrate, mainly lymphocytic, of stria vascularis.
    Illustration courtesy Lindsay and Hemenway, *Ann Otol, 63*:754, 1954.

ologic alterations are essentially the same as in mumps. In the active stage lymphomononuclear infiltrate is observed, with the appearance of multinucleated forms (Lindsay and Hemenway, 1954).

    Labyrinthitis of influenzal origin occurs in relation to, or shortly following, upper respiratory infection. The findings are like those in the previously described viral infections.

    In an active stage of viral labyrinthitis the capillary endothelium, especially of the stria vascularis, is swollen and proliferated, and there may be micropetechiae with local inflammatory response (Snow, 1973). As has been indicated, the labyrinthine injury is type IV (Scheibe); viral infections are one of the main causes of cochleosaccular degeneration (Schuknecht, Igarashi and Gacek, 1965). Ectopic bone formation is not characteristic.

Central nervous system involvement with viruses represents an important segment of neuropathology. The few available specific auditory pathway findings are overshadowed by those in the labyrinth in those cases in which deafness is an individually appreciable manifestation.

PARASITIC INFECTIONS

Toxoplasmosis

Toxoplasmosis was mentioned previously as a congenital disorder.

Syphilis

In syphilis, auditory lesions are noteworthy (Dublin, 1967; Karmody and Schuknecht, 1966; Paparella and Capps, 1973; Perlman, 1973; Igarashi, 1972; Wilson, 1940). About 40 percent of congenital luetics complain of hearing loss; one third of these are children. The disease may appear as a part of the secondary stage in the first two years of life, or tertiary from ages eight to twenty. Onset tends to be sudden; it is characteristically sensorineural with flat audiometric curve and almost always is bilateral. There is osteitis and periostitis with a gummatous pattern, the small blood vessels showing obliterative endothelial proliferation. Miliary gummas may appear throughout the spiral ganglion. The foci of destruction are replaced with fibrous tissue, followed by new bone formation that may be obliterative. Endolymphatic hydrops develops, the basis of which is not clear; the disorder may be symptomatically indistinguishable from Meniere's syndrome. The organ of Corti degenerates. There is variable degeneration of the spiral ganglion and auditory nerve (*see* Figures 51 A & B *and* 52 A & B).

Loss of hearing is an important feature of acquired syphilis; it is a frequent accompaniment of tabetic amaurosis (Wilson, 1940), involvement of the eighth nerve being second to that of the optic. Histologically the nerve shows demyelination together with lymphocytic and plasma cell infiltrate as in optic neuritis. Representing

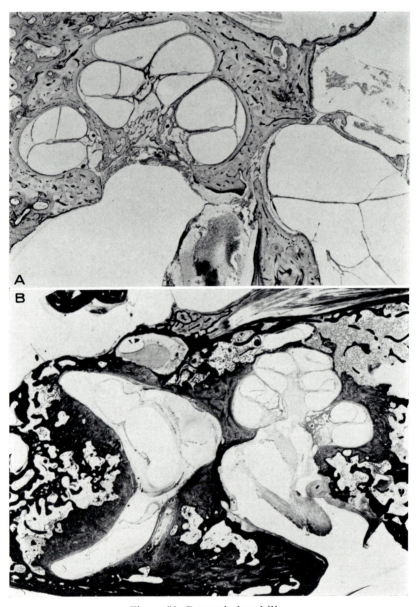

Figure 51. Congenital syphilis.

Figure 51A. Internal auditory meatus is lined by thickened dura and contains herniated cerebellum. There is endolymphatic hydrops. Very few spiral

a notable segment of neuropathology, the central portions of the auditory pathway are variably involved along with the rest of the brain in the processes of meningoencephalitis, vascular occlusion and gummatous inflammation, with similarly variable effects on the integrative and associational functions. Detailed, specific auditory pathway reviews are needed. Syphilis is an excellent example of the need for properly-controlled, simultaneous, full-auditory pathway studies in hearing disorders.

IMMUNE DISORDERS

The Lupus-Polyarteritis-Rheumatic Group of Disorders

The auditory pathway shares in the involvement of the nervous system in the lupus-polyarteritis-rheumatic disorder. Data pertaining to the perceptive as well as the integrative features of hearing are needed.

Cogan's Syndrome

Cogan's syndrome (Schuknecht, 1974) consists of vestibulo-auditory symptoms in association with nonsyphilitic interstitial keratitis. There may be sudden onset of vertigo, tinnitus, nausea and vomiting associated with rapidly-developing sensorineural hearing loss. General pathologic findings are those of systemic necrotizing angiitis of polyarteritis type. Temporal bone study has revealed endolymphatic hydrops with marked distortion and fenestration of the vestibular membrane. New bone formation was found within the thickened round window membrane. There was degeneration of the organ of Corti and cochlear neurons, most severe in the basal turn (Wolff, Bernhard, Tsutsumi, et al., 1965).

---

ganglion neurons are present.

Figure 51B. Extensive erosion of the otic capsule and of the margins of the internal auditory meatus has occurred. Spaces in the otic capsule are filled with highly cellular marrow-like tissue or loose connective tissue containing round cells.

Illustration courtesy Schuknecht (Karmody and Schuknecht), *Arch Otolaryngol, 83*:18, 1966, copyright American Medical Association. Figure 51B was originally courtesy Dr. Luzius Ruedi.

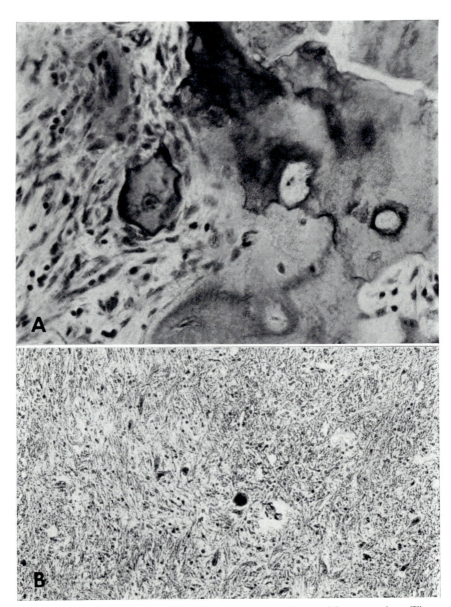

Figure 52A. Congenital syphilis, high power of a focus of bony erosion. The chronic inflammatory tissue contained in the osseous spaces includes lymphocytes and plasma cells, and a multinucleated foreign body giant cell is seen at upper left.

Figure 52B. Neurosyphilis. Medial dorsal olivary nucleus (slanting down from upper left toward low center) shows severe neuronal loss with general tissue rarefaction and gliosis. So severe involvement of this nucleus may not neccessarily be expected characteristically or regularly.

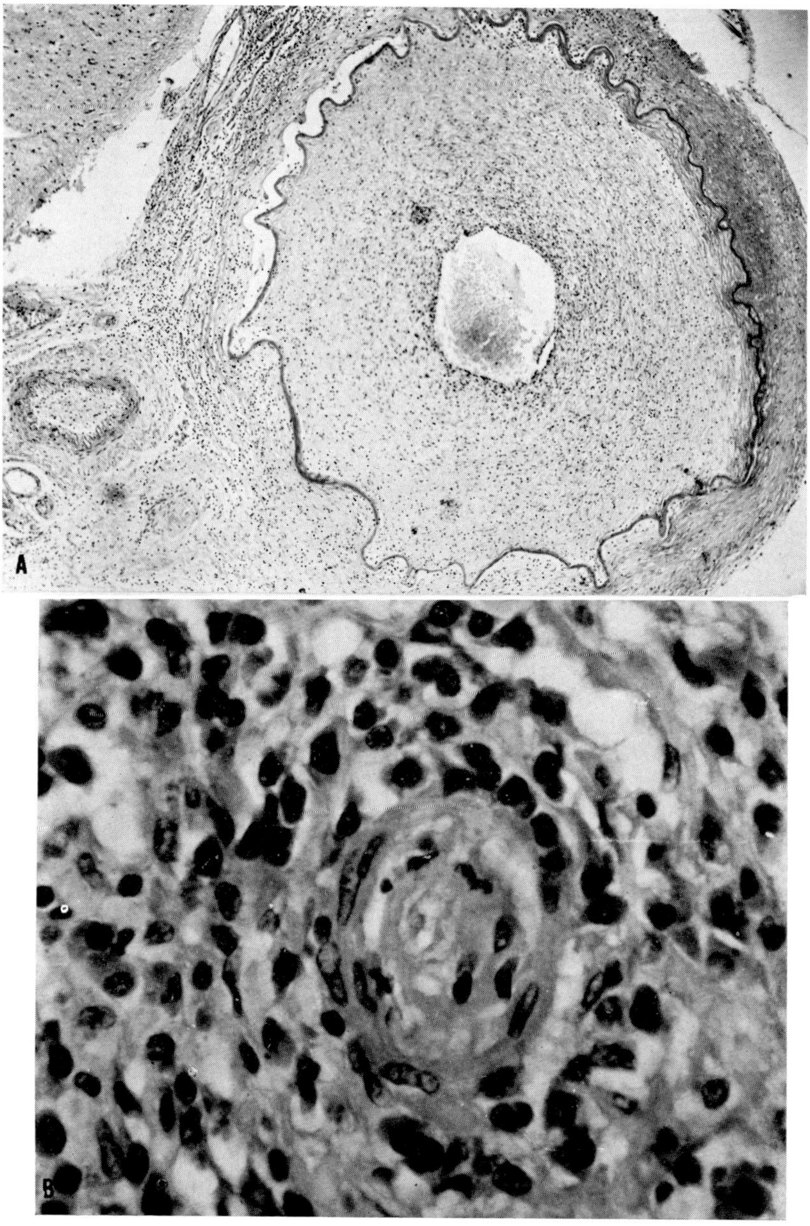

Figure 53A. Syphilitic endarteritis, meninges of medulla.
Figure 53B. Basic histopathologic structure of gumma showing obliterative endarteritis with infiltration of lymphocytes and plasma cells in and about the vessel.

Illustrations from Dublin, *Fundamentals of Neuropathology*, Ed. II, Charles C Thomas, 1967.

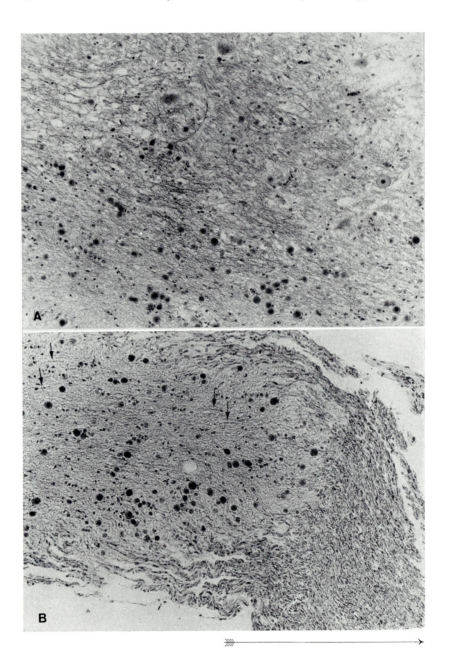

Disseminated Sclerosis

The degree to which hearing is affected in disseminated sclerosis is estimated quite variably, ranging from seldom if ever (Wilson, 1940) to frequent (von Leden, 1948) to the great majority (Noffsinger, Olsen, Carhart et al., 1972). Pure tone audiometry may not reveal the aberration; more subtle audiometric techniques may be required to show hearing abnormality (Le Zak and Selhub, 1966; Noffsinger, Olsen, Carhart et al., 1972). The audiogram may be flat, with full-range loss, or high frequency. The disturbance of hearing, like other manifestations of disseminated sclerosis, may be transitory, at least in a developing stage, and is quite variable.

The basic pathogenic process is one of destruction of myelin by antibody developed against antigen formed by union of myelin with the projected virus. Central nervous system involvement is protean, and integrative processes may be affected commensurately. There is proliferation of lymphocytes and macrophages in white matter undergoing demyelination. In late stages there is absence of myelin with increase of glia, the latter tending to be arranged in dense bands.

The peripheral hearing organ is characteristically spared (Dix, 1965; Hallpike, 1967). Sensorineural hearing loss may result from involvement of the cochlear nucleus and/or trapezoid body; the VIIIth nerve is seldom affected (Noffsinger, Olsen, Carhart et al., 1972). Clinical manifestations reflect the involvement also of higher nuclear centers and pathways from the brain stem to the cortex.

Figure 54. Neurosyphilis.
Figure 54A. Involvement of hilum of cochlear nerve (lower left) with production of corpora amylacea. Margin of superior ventral cochlear nucleus shows injury (upper right); a few spheroid cells survive, variably well preserved.
Figure 54B. Degeneration of cochlear nerve, luxol fast blue, yellow filter. The central (glial) portion of the nerve (to left) is severely demyelinated; the few surviving myelin sheaths are seen as short, slightly dark, delicate threads (arrows indicate examples). Numerous corpora amylacea have accumulated on the central side of the lamina cribrosa. The peripheral (neurolemmal) segment on lower right is also degenerated as shown by a porous and slightly uneven appearance.

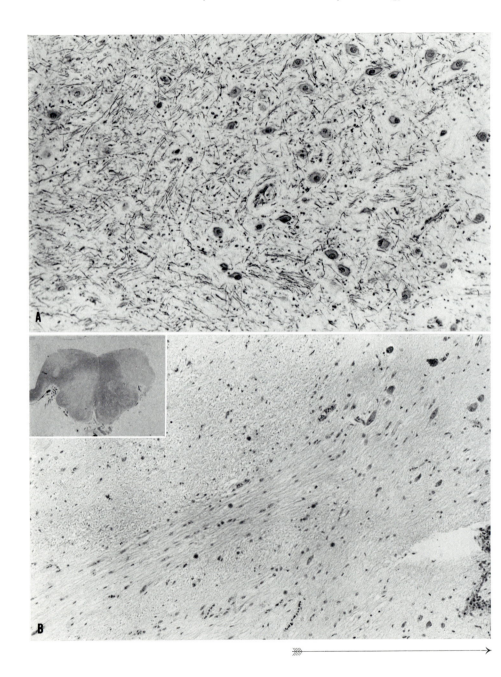

Relation to Meniere's Syndrome

Allergy appears to play a part in the pathogenesis of Meniere's syndrome.

Encephalomyeloneuropathy in Neoplastic Diseases

The encephalopathy and neuropathy occurring in association with neoplastic diseases may include the structures of the auditory pathway (Schuknecht, 1974).

Figure 55A. Transverse view of right superior ventral cochlear nucleus, Bodian stain, from a case of disseminated sclerosis in which there was no apparent involvement of cochlear nuclear complex. Well-preserved spheroid cells are seen on the right, and on the left, fibers of the trapezoid body sweep diagonally downward to left.

Figure 55B. Section from same location as in Figure 55A from another case of disseminated sclerosis in which there was involvement of the cochlear nucleus and trapezoid body. A few remnant spheroid cells appear at upper right. A band of gliosis extends down across center to the left. Inset shows large foci of demyelination in a section of medulla from the same case (luxol fast blue stain), one of the foci including the right cochlear nucleus and trapezoid complex. This type of lesion can produce unilateral sensorineural hearing loss equivalent to that resulting from demyelination of the cochlear nerve.

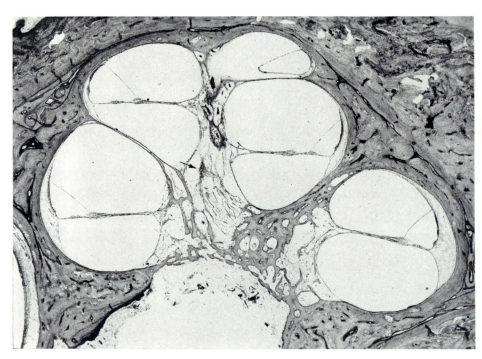

Figure 56. Encephalomyeloneuropathy on an immune basis in association with anaplastic (oat cell) carcinoma of lung; widespread nervous system involvement was found including severe loss of cochlear neurons. A few fibers which survived were thought to be efferent (arrow). Organ of Corti was found atrophic in the basal 9 mm. There was also degeneration of the cochlear nerve and nucleus. Illustration courtesy Schuknecht, *Pathology of the Ear.* Harvard University Press, 1974.

Chapter 6 _____

INJURIES

_____

CLOSED HEAD INJURIES

CONCUSSION IMPLIES THE INTERRUPTION of function in absence of structural change. It appears likely, however, that injury, however mild, that produces symptoms is attended by pathologic alteration of some form and degree. The auditory pathway may be affected. Blows to the head send waves of force through the tissues; this is transmitted to the inner ear in the form of high intensity vibratory energy. Sensorineural hearing loss can occur in the resulting labyrinthine concussion (Hough, 1973; Igarashi, 1972; Proctor, Gurdjian and Webster, 1956; Ward, 1969; Schuknecht, 1969). The loss is greater for tones between 3000 and 8000 cps. Outer hair cells are involved first and may be injured or lost, followed by inner hair cells. With increase of degree of stress, injury may extend to complete disappearance of the organ of Corti in the related zone; in such cases the cochlear neurons have been found to be involved, although less severely (Schuknecht, 1969).

The cochlear nuclear complex and higher centers also may be affected in this state of *commotio cerebri*. In addition to changes of nerve cells, some degree of congestion and edema also tends to be present. Clinical cerebral concussion is accompanied also by chemical changes such as the appearance in cerebrospinal fluid of acetylcholine, serotonin and nucleic acid breakdown products; the blood-brain barrier may show diminished integrity.

More severe degrees of intracranial injury may be encountered. Closed head injury may result in complete destruction of all major functional units within the temporal bone (Hough, 1973). This applies equally to the central nervous system where the most devastating brain injury may occur with no outward evidence of violence. The lesions that may occur include edema; hemorrhage occuring within the brain or in extradural, intradural, subdural, or subarachnoid location; laceration; contusion; and cranial nerve injury. Such lesions tend to occur in combinations. The structure of the central part of the auditory pathway will be involved variably along with other brain tissues. Traumatic pathogenic mechanisms per se are complicated by accompanying anoxia. Specific auditory study is needed in cases of head injury, especially where audiograms have been performed.

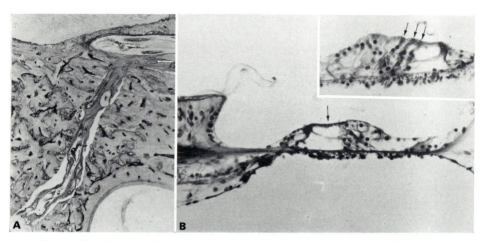

Figure 57A. Fracture involving the wall of the otic capsule. New bone has been formed within the fracture line.

Figure 57B. Loss of hair cells has occurred as a residual of head injury (arrow). Inset shows normal hair cells (arrows) for comparison.

Illustrations courtesy Schuknecht, *Pathology of the Ear,* Harvard University Press, 1974.

FRACTURES

If the physical stress sustained is sufficiently severe, skull fracture may occur; the temporal bone may be involved (Hough, 1973; Igarashi, 1972; Proctor, Gurdjian and Webster, 1956; Lindsay, 1973a; Schuknecht, 1969). Fractures of the petrous bone may be longitudinal, transverse or mixed; the latter variety is common, pure longitudinal or transverse fracture being encountered less often, and some degree of comminution being the rule. Longitudinal fractures result from transversely-directed blows to the temporoparietal region. The fracture tends to pass around the hard bone of the otic capsule; the external and middle ear receive most of the damage, with conductive hearing loss. Fronto-occipital force tends to produce transverse fractures of the petrous bone, frequently by incorporation into a posterior basal fracture. The labyrinth is damaged more often in the transverse variety. Small fissures may be seen; they require exclusion of artifact. Where reaction of connective and vascular tissues and/or bone is observed, especially if the newly-formed tissue is interposed within the fracture line, the ante mortem nature of the finding is supported. In transverse fractures the vestibule and/or cochlea tend to be opened, with creation of a communication with the internal auditory canal. The eighth cranial nerve may be injured. Either or both windows may be ruptured. Hearing loss is abrupt and total, and prognosis is unfavorable. Injury of the tissues of the cochlear membranous labyrinth is widespread and severe. Hemorrhages occur within the cochlea. This, especially, is followed by proliferation of connective tissue, followed in turn by obliterative ossification. Endosteal and periosteal bone can and will react, but the endochondral layer remains inert, healing only with connective tissue, with no evidence of osseous repair; fractures tend to persist ununited. In such cases infection within the tympanic cavity may invade the labyrinth.

Skull fractures may represent a part of head injuries affecting the central portion of the auditory pathway. The specific effect on hearing is not as pointed as it is in the peripheral hearing organ even though the auditory centers manifestly participate in the general effects of injury.

ACOUSTIC TRAUMA

Acoustic trauma may be a complex disorder in that different forms of noise may cause different types of damage (Engström, Ades and Bredberg, 1970). In injury from acoustic overstimulation (Igarashi, 1972; Spoendlin and Brun, 1973; Ward, 1973; Ward and Duvall, 1971) the factors of intensity and duration of exposure are superimposed. A single blast of short duration, if sufficiently intense, may produce loss of sensorineural hearing, apparently by excessive movement of the basilar membrane. At the other end of the

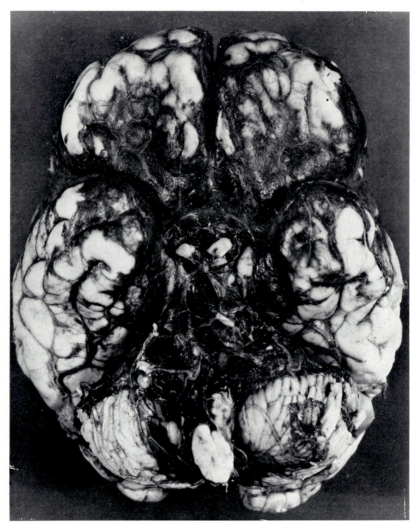

Figure 58. Traumatic subarachnoid hemorrhage in an adult. Cochlear nerves and brain stem are included notably in the involvement. Illustration from Dublin, *Fundamentals of Neuropathology,* Ed. II, Charles C Thomas, 1967.

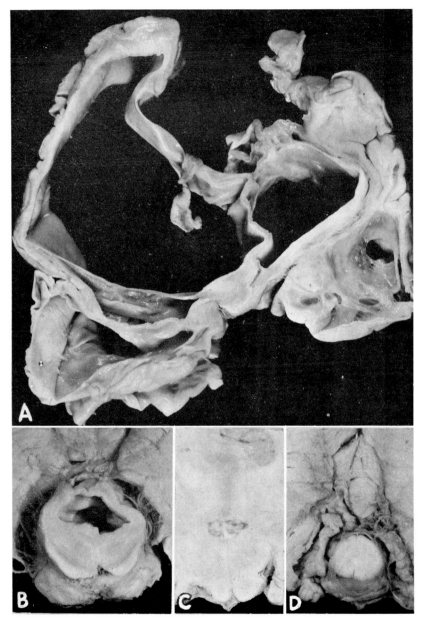

Figure 59. Status postbirth injury with organization of hemorrhages which occurred about the base, leading to hydrocephalus. Auditory information not available. (A) Dilated lateral ventricles and cerebral atrophy. (B) Dilated aqueduct. (C) Internal or superior view of obstruction of outflow of fourth ventricle. (D) Adhesions about the medulla and pons. Illustration from Dublin, *Fundamentals of Neuropathology,* Ed. II, Charles C Thomas, 1967.

spectrum is the effect of less intense but sustained and/or persistently repeated sound, resulting in high frequency loss similar to that of presbycusis, maximal at around 4000 cps, representing the middle portion of the basal turn. One wonders whether the hearing loss thought to be a part of the aging process actually represents the cumulative result of chronic exposure to sound. Contrariwise, one can rarely be certain in full degree of a pure case of long-term acoustic injury; there is inevitable contamination with the features of senescence. The possibility of biochemical changes is to be considered as a factor in the production of deafness by chronic exposure to excessive sound (Ward, 1973). Intense experimental tonal stimulation leads to increase of endolymphatic sodium and decrease of potassium, with return to original levels following discontinuation of the tonal stimulus (Suga, Nakashima and Snow, 1970).

In acoustic trauma, as in injury from some other causes, the outer hair cells are affected first, followed, as the degree of stress increases, by inner hair cells and supporting elements, leading to destruction of the entire organ of Corti. The supporting cells have been found to be affected less often in human material (Igarashi, 1972). The range of intensity found to induce pathologic changes experimentally is 90 to 130 db (Spoendlin and Brun, 1973). Degeneration of ganglion cells will occur regional to that of the organ of Corti; it depends on the state of preservation of the supporting elements. The stria vascularis appears comparatively unaltered.

Permanent threshold alteration results from loss, not of outer, but of inner hair cells; this feature supports the theory that the outer hair cells are not essential to, and serve a purpose other than, acuity of hearing (Ward and Duvall, 1971). The greater effect on outer hair cells in exposure to excessive sound could result from the more apparent firm attachment of hairs of outer hair cells to the tectorial membrane (Kimura, 1966) (*see* Figure 61 A & B).

The first and most subtle effects of acoustic overstimulation (experimental in guinea pigs) are in the form of blebs appearing on the ends of hairs of outer hair cells (Lim and Melnick, 1971). This alteration, which is beyond the reasonable reach of light micros-

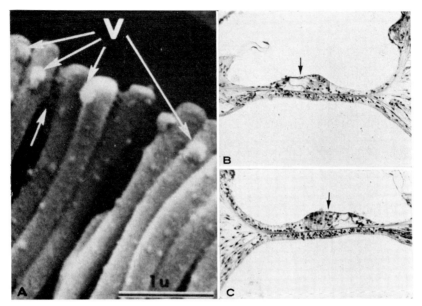

Figure 60. Acoustic trauma.
Figure 60A (Experimental). Bleb formation on ends of hairs of outer hair cells. Illustration courtesy Lim, *Arch Otolaryngol, 94*:294, 1971, copyright American Medical Association.
Figure 60B. Severe hearing loss at 4000 to 8000 Hz in a boilermaker and steam fitter is reflected in loss of external hair cells (arrow) in the 2 to 15 mm (from base of cochlea) zone. In Figure 60C, normal hair cells (arrow) are shown for comparison. Illustration courtesy Schuknecht, *Pathology of the Ear,* Harvard University Press, 1974.

copy, could interrupt the hearing mechanism at the hair level. These blebs are found also on normal hairs, but in notably fewer numbers. They appear throughout all turns of the cochlea but are more numerous in the region of predicted maximal displacement of the basilar membrane. Intracellular alterations consist of nuclear pyknosis and cytoplasmic vacuolization, the latter involving endoplasmic reticulum. As the changes progress, the hair cells disintegrate; the spaces thus formed are filled with scars formed chiefly by phalangeal processes. The cuticular lamina, normally a firm plate, becomes softened.

Constriction of nutrient capillaries occurs following exposure to

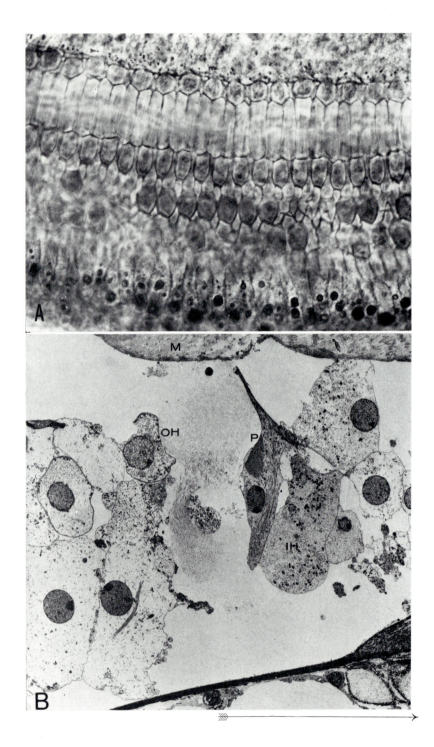

excessive noise (Hawkins, 1971; Lipscomb and Roettger, 1973; Ward, 1973). Swelling of endothelium results in blockage to the passage of erythrocytes. In this way exposure to noise may accelerate the process of devascularization of the membranous labyrinth that begins in fetal life (Hawkins, Johnsson and Preston, 1972). Endolymphatic oxygen tension is reduced in acoustic overstimulation (Hawkins, 1971).

Ultrasound

Ultrasound affects the outer hair cells primarily; with increased stress, inner hair cells may be involved. If the supporting cells are injured, hair cells will not survive. Early, there is spreading and disarray of stereocilia. Cytoplasmic changes include nuclear swelling and granularity of cytoplasm (Crysdale and Stahle, 1972). Injury of the stria vascularis has been observed (Sugar, Engström and Stahle, 1972).

BAROTRAUMA

Rupture of the round window membrane may be observed in association with sudden deafness; there may be history of recent diving (Edmonds, Freeman and Tonkin, 1974; Pang, 1974; Pullen, 1972). Fistula may develop. Healing tends to occur spontaneously within a few weeks; in some cases, surgical closure has enhanced recovery from the hearing loss.

Auditory tissues may be included in involvement in cases of the bends where too-rapid decompression results in air embolism of branches of the labyrinthine artery (Pang, 1974). Treatment with inhalation of hyperbaric oxygen has been recommended for cases of sudden sensorineural hearing loss where the basis appears to be vascular, especially if the condition is refractory to admin-

---

Figure 61. Experimental acoustic trauma, guinea pig.
Figure 61A. Surface preparation showing loss of outer hair cells at bottom, increasing toward left. Illustration courtesy Hawkins, *Ann Otol, 80*:903, 1971.
Figure 61B. Electron microphotograph showing disruption of organ of Corti. (M) Tectorial membrane. (P) Pillar. (OH) Outer hair cell. (IH) Inner hair cell. Illustration courtesy Spoendlin and Brun, *Acta Otolaryngol, 75*:220, 1973.

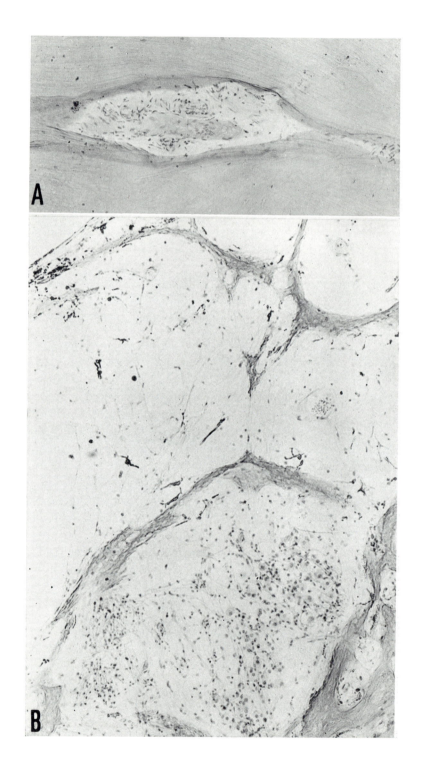

istration of vasodilators (Pang, 1974). Interference with blood supply to the brain stem (cochlear nucleus) is quite as deserving of such consideration. Whole-auditory pathway studies are needed.

LASER IRRADIATION

Laser injury has been studied experimentally in mice. Severe cochlear damage was found with occurrence of hemorrhages. Primary injury to sensory end-organs was irregular and inconstant (Keleman, Laor and Klein, 1967). Injury of the stria vascularis has been observed (Sugar, Engström and Stahle, 1972).

PENETRATING IRRADIATION

The inner ear is exposed with impunity to penetrating radiation in the treatment of malignant disease, the latter overshadowing possible auditory loss. The labyrinth would appear to be relatively resistant. Variable hearing loss has been reported, extending to total loss in some cases (Gamble, Peterson and Chandler, 1968). Osteoporosis resembling that of the idiopathic type has been observed (Jørgensen and Kristensen, 1966). Most experimental observations have been those of the acute results of total body irradiation. Auditory changes were found on the administration of 3000 rads or more. Opinion varies as to prime sensitivity of stria vascularis (Gamble, Peterson and Chandler, 1968) versus hair cells, especially outer hair cells of the two basal turns (guinea pig) (Winther, 1970).

The neuroglial parenchyma of the central nervous system is relatively insensitive to penetrating radiation. Effects are produced mainly through injury of blood vessels, resulting in focal destruction of brain tissue. Hyaline thickening and necrosis of the vessel walls, especially of arterioles, is noteworthy, and amyloid may be deposited. Specific auditory pathway studies are needed.

Figure 62. Effects of deep irradiation.
Figure 62A. Hyaline sclerosis of arteriole, otic capsule.
Figure 62B. Estimated 40 percent loss of spiral ganglion neurons (lower part of field).

MEDICINAL INTOXICATION

An unfortunate complication that may follow the administration of various medicinal substances is loss of hearing. This is true notably regarding antibiotics (Brummett, Himes, Saine *et al.*, 1972, Engström, Ades and Andersson, 1966; Engström and Kohonen, 1965; Gonzales, Miller and Wasilewski, 1972; Igarashi, 1972; Kaku, Farmer and Hudson, 1973; Kohonen, 1965; Logan, Prazma, Thomas *et al.*, 1974, Mendelsohn and Katzenberg, 1972; Meuwissen and Robinsin, 1967; Quick, 1973; Saito and Daly, 1971). The sensory epithelium is notably affected. The balance between cochlear and renal effects of some of the principal agents has been tabulated (Meuwissen and Robinson, 1967):

	Effects On	
	Cochlea	*Kidney*
Streptomycin	+	+
Dihydrostreptomycin	++++	+
Neomycin	++++	+++
Kanamycin	+++	+++
Vancomycin	+++	+
Viomycin	++	+
Framycetin	++++	
Gentamycin		++
Colistin	+	++

Tobramycin also may be toxic (Brummett, Himes, Saine *et al.*, 1972). The detailed effects of the various antibiotics have been listed (Quick, 1973).

The basic clinical auditory manifestation is high-frequency hearing loss occurring especially in association with renal insufficiency; failure of excretion of antibiotics enhances and prolongs the toxic effect. In keeping with the high-frequency loss, degeneration is found in the organ of Corti, usually most severe in the basal turn, progressing toward the apex. As in certain other conditions, the outer hair cells are especially vulnerable. Injury of inner hair cells follows. The earliest histologic sign of injury is the disarrangement of the W pattern of the stereocilia (Gonzales, Miller, and

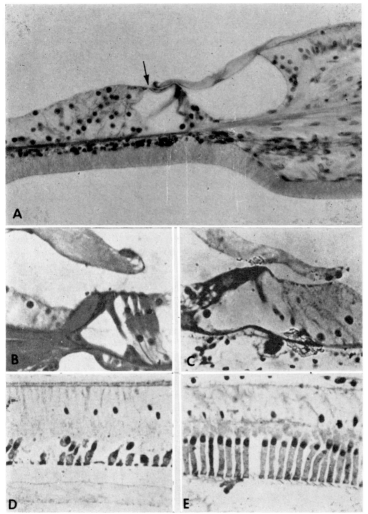

Figure 63A. Kanamycin deafness. Organ of Corti is slightly collapsed. All hair cells are missing (arrow). Dense eosinophilic precipitate appears beneath basement membrane .Illustration courtesy Igarashi in Minckler (Ed.): Pathology of the Nervous System, copyright McGraw-Hill, 1972.

Figures 63B and C. Ethacrynic acid toxicity, cat. Normal organ of Corti on left for comparison. On right, organ of Corti shows injury, especially to the outer hair cells. Figures 63 D and E. The same, tangential sections.

Figures 63B, C, D and E after Mathog (with Thomas and Hudson), *Arch Otolaryngol, 92:*7, 1970, copyright American Medical Association.

Wasilewski, 1972). Intracellular changes follow. The ultimate of injury is disappearance of the organ of Corti. The places occupied previously by the sensory cells are filled with phalangeal scars. The state of the nerve fibers is somewhat parallel with that of the supporting cells.

The toxic effects on hearing appear to be mediated through chemical mechanisms. The respiratory activity of the cochlea, notably of outer hair cells and stria vascularis, is disturbed (Kaku, Farmer and Hudson, 1973). Decline of electric potential is observed. Adenosine triphosphatase may be decreased in stria vascularis, thus interfering with the transport mechanism (Mendelsohn and Katzenberg, 1972). The energy supply of the sensory cells may be impeded (Meuwissen and Robinson, 1967).

Significant histopathologic changes of the auditory brain stem nuclei were not found following administration of streptomycin and dihydrostreptomycin (cat) (McGee and Olszewski, 1962). This was in comparison with characteristic lesions of the organ of Corti in the same animals. Nothing like the toxic effects produced on the peripheral hearing organ by the administration of antibiotics has been observed in the central part of the auditory pathway.

Quinine and salicylates produce disturbances of hearing. The effects appear to be reversible (Igarashi, 1972; Perez De Moura and Hayden, 1968).

Chapter 7 ──────────────────────────────

TUMORS

────────────────────────────────────

REGIONS OF INVOLVEMENT

THE PETROUS PYRAMID is not often the site of primary origin of neoplasms, and, indeed, tends to resist secondary involvement by invasion. The acoustic nerve is an important situation of primary neoplasia. Intracranial tumors of the various histologic types, whose detailed account is somewhat beyond the scope of the present discussion (Dublin, 1967), may occupy the temporal lobe, auditory radiation, posterior thalamus, midbrain, pons and medulla, involving the corresponding portions of the auditory pathway. Except for the cochlear nucleus and contiguous portion of the trapezoid body, the central auditory representation is bilateral; in cases of more centrally situated pathologic alteration, there naturally will be some variable effect on the more integrative aspects of hearing, but these are not easily defined in terms of concise localization of involvement. This is borne out by the absence, to date, of reliable data on the boundaries of the auditory cortical areas, despite all of the study, in the past, of the very considerable available pathologic material. Intrinsic involvement of the brain stem so situated as to cause unilateral hearing loss is liable to be attended by interference with the vital processes to a degree rendering the auditory disability comparatively unimportant, assuming that meaningful neurologic and audiometric evaluation can be conducted.

Opinion differs regarding the effect on hearing of increase of intracranial pressure. No correlation was found between increased pressure and state of hearing (Hansen, 1968a) ; some degree of hearing loss was encountered frequently, about one-half sensorineural, in general exhibiting flat audiometric curves, and improvement occurring in a significant number of cases following relief of pressure (Saxena, Tandon, Sinha, *et al.*, 1969) .

The main alteration of hearing by neoplasms is by compromise of the cochlear neurons, notably as represented in the cochlear nerve. This may occur within the internal acoustic meatus or subarachnoid space, or in the cerebellopontine recess. The cochlear nucleus and adjacent brain stem tissue may be injured by growths in the latter situation.

The cerebellopontine recess is formed by the junction of cerebellum, pons and medulla. Clinical manifestations of tumors in this location (Schuknecht, 1974) include those of cochlear nerve injury, i.e. tinnitus and loss of hearing; increased intracranial pressure, including headache and papilledema; cerebellar symptoms, as incoordination, especially of the lower limbs; involvement of adjacent cranial nerves, V and VII earlier, and VI, IX and X later; and, in the presence of severe compression of the brain stem, pyramidal signs. The percentile incidence of histologic types of cerebellopontine recess tumors has been found as neurofibroma, 78; meningioma, 6.5; epidermoid cyst, 6.3 (Gonzalez-Rivella, 1947); gliomas extending from within the lateral recess of the fourth ventricle also deserve individual mention. Other tumor types include arachnoid cyst, aneurysm, and vascular and connective tissue tumors, benign and malignant (Hitselberger and Gardner, 1968; Schuknecht, 1974) . Granuloma may act as neoplasm. Metastatic carcinoma doubtless occurs more often than is usually thought, but as a part of multiple metastases, and the effects of the latter tend to overshadow the acoustic manifestations per se. The cochlear nerve may be involved by the subarachnoid dissemination of a malignant neoplasm such as an anaplastic glioma; such involvement may extend into the internal auditory meatus (Nager, 1967). Extrameningeal invasion by, or metastasis from, an intracranial neoplasm, however, occurs but rarely, and then almost solely from sarcoma (Dublin, 1944a) . The meningovascular barrier is almost absolute against passage by glioma; in almost every case in which such a tumor has been reported extending outside the meninges, the barrier has been broken by surgical incision, injury, infection or other, similar process.

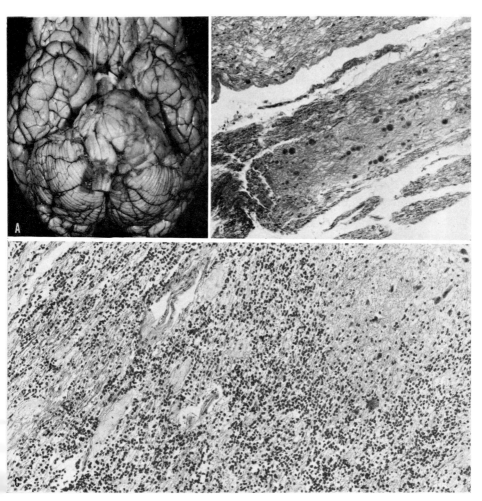

Figure 64A. Tumor composed of astrocytes and polar glioblasts in girl, aged ten, infiltrating, destroying and expanding the brain stem with bulging of tumor into cerebellopontine recess. Illustration from Dublin, *Fundamentals of Neuropathology*, Ed. II, Charles C Thomas, 1967.

Figure 64B. Same case showing degeneration of the compressed cochlear nerve.

Figure 64C. Infiltration of cochlear nerve and superior ventral cochlear nucleus by cerebral glioma that has spread through the subarachnoid space. A few residual, degenerated spheroid cells are seen at upper right.

NEUROFIBROMA

The stated incidence of histologic types of neoplasms tends to be inconstant owing to inevitable factors of selection in different institutions; however, neurofibroma accounts for roughly 9 to 10 percent of intracranial tumors (Schuknecht, 1974) and four fifths of tumors of the cerebellopontine recess (Gonzalez-Revilla, 1947). Two thirds of subjects are female. Age peak is at thirty-five to forty years.

The great majority of intracranial neurofibromas is acoustic (Igarashi, 1972; Schuknecht, 1974) ; a few such tumors arise from the fifth cranial nerve, rarely from the third, seventh or ninth (Mountjoy, Dolan and McCabe, 1974) to twelfth (Nager, 1969a). Most eighth nerve tumors are of the vestibular division, and in every case, the peripheral or neurolemmal portion. Four percent of acoustic neurofibromas are bilateral, mainly as a manifestation of von Recklinghausen's disease, as are those tumors of glossopharyngeal and vagus nerves and motor nerve roots; such cases are genetic in basis and appear to constitute a separate disorder.

The symptoms of acoustic neurofibroma, together with the histopathologic lesions that mediate them, may vary considerably; they include especially tinnitus and hearing loss. Audiometric features have been outlined (Liden, 1969; Johnson, 1969). Impairment of speech discrimination tends to be greater than would be expected on a basis of the pure tone threshold. This is in keeping with the finding that only a small proportion, i.e. 25 percent, of cochlear neurons will suffice for pure tone perception, but a more substantial complement is needed for the more complex and more centrally-based processes involved in speech discrimination. Loudness recruitment is thought to be characteristically absent, but may occur as a secondary effect of impairment of labyrinthine blood supply. Atypical cases of Meniere's syndrome may be distinguished from acoustic neurofibroma with difficulty.

The effect of neurofibroma on hearing may be contributed to in some degree by biochemical changes in the inner ear fluids (Silverstein, 1973; Silverstein, Naufal and Belal, 1973), the most striking of which is increase of protein. In the presence of smaller neurofibromas, cerebrospinal fluid protein may be less than 50 mg/

100 ml, making this feature of commensurately limited value for diagnosis in relatively early cases. Diagnostic labyrinthotomy offers potential value under certain circumstances. Because of the occurrence of further sensorineural hearing loss in one third of the cases after the procedure, the latter should be performed only when no serviceable hearing is present in the ear being tested (Silverstein, 1973).

Acoustic neurofibromas, most of them growing within the inner acoustic meatus, impinge on fibers of the cochlear nerve, injuring them variably; the neuronal complement of the spiral ganglion is depleted commensurately. Ischemic effects on the inner ear, generally, may be produced by compression of the labyrinthine vessels. As the tumor enlarges it may erode the osseous wall of the meatus; in due course it may grow out through the aperture of the meatus into the cerebellopontine recess, or enlarge *in situ* in the recess if the tumor arose *de novo* in that position, and neurologic manifestations are produced accordingly. Infrequently, the growth of the neurofibroma may be confined entirely within the temporal bone. The modiolus and/or vestibule may be invaded, and, rarely, the tumor arises within the cochlea (Gussen 1971a; Karlan, Basek and Potter, 1972). Small, asymptomatic tumors on occasion are found incidentally (Leonard and Talbot, 1970) (*see* Figures 66 A & B).

Grossly, the tumor nodule is well-circumscribed, usually encapsulated, sometimes lobulated, the latter especially with reference to the intracranial portion of a tumor originating within the acoustic meatus. The cut surface is firm, fleshy to fibrous and pink to pale, tannish gray. There may be cystic cavitation. Hemorrhagic and lipoid degeneration impart red and yellow coloration respectively (*see* Figures 67 A & B).

Microscopically, the four elements of the nerve fiber (sheath of Schwann, axis cylinder, myelin sheath and endometrum) appear to a point where the resulting tumor is properly referred to inclusively as neurofibroma. The various other terms which have been employed, including schwannoma, neurolemmoma and perineural fibroblastoma, are limited in scope and do not recognize the essential full participation of the components of the nerve fiber; they may properly be used in denoting main tissue type or component

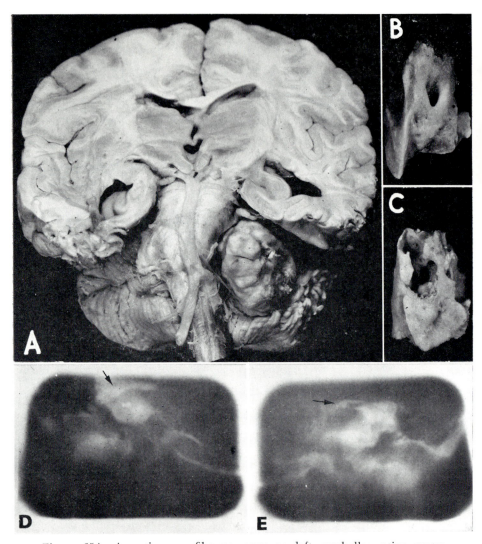

Figure 65A. Acoustic neurofibroma grow as left cerebollopontine recess tumor with displacement and compression of adjacent structures.

Figure 65B. Normal right inner acoustic meatus.

Figure 65C. Left inner acoustic meatus showing destruction of the osseous wall.

Figure 65D,E. Tomograms of inner ear from a case of acoustic neurofibroma.

Figure 65D. Shows normal roof of inner acoustic meatus (arrow).

Figure 65E. Roof of meatus eroded (arrow).

Roentgenograms courtesy Dr. Mansfield F. W. Smith.

of a tumor. The recognition of histologic subtypes offers no prognostic advantage.

The active nutrient and reparative capacity of the nurolemma is reasonably reflected in the leading participation of Schwann cells in the majority of neurofibromas (Skinner, 1929). These slender, elongated cells tend to appear in a somewhat whorled pattern, frequently arranged in palisades separated by acellular foci frequently traversed by axis cylinders. The latter may also be found irregularly throughout the tumor; they can be demonstrated with silver impregnation, especially with protargol, the latter introducing less of interfering staining of reticulum than do the compound ammoniacal silver solutions. Counterstaining as in the Masson trichrome method (Dublin, 1944b) adds the visualization of myelin sheaths. These can be found in most neurofibromas. Some of the tumors are composed appreciably or even preponderantly of fully-developed myelinated nerve fibers, although in other cases the myelin appears less frequently and in attenuated form; outfoldings of the sheaths have been observed (Schulz and Hildering, 1970). Endoneurium participates variably in neurofibroma. Collagen may accordingly be deposited in considerable amounts; it may be contributed to by organizing fibroblasts, representing a product of degeneration. Rarefaction similarly may be seen to a maximum of cavitation. The hemorrhage and fatty degeneration seen grossly are observed microscopically, with the appearance of blood pigment and lipoid-containing macrophages. Ischemia tends to produce enlarged, darkly and homogenously staining nuclei. Two histologic types have been recognized on the basis of compact versus loose cellular organization, Antoni types A and B. The difference is appreciably accountable as a process of degenerative loosening of the tissue; the two categories have no practical import and do not deserve further consideration. Malignant forms of acoustic neurofibroma are encountered scarcely if ever.

An unusual tumor of the cochlear nerve has been encountered, appearing to arise from the lamina cribrosa (membrana perforata) and tending to reproduce its basic fibrous sieve-like structure (Fig. 66).

In acoustic neurofibroma, degeneration of the organ of Corti is observed variably, resulting largely from compromise of the laby-

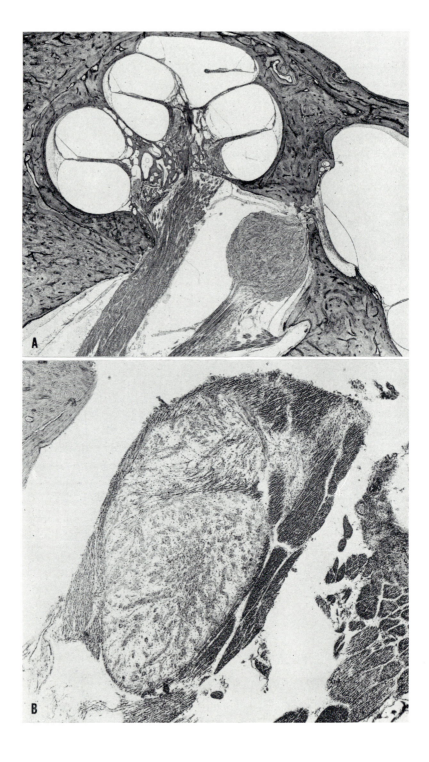

rinthine vessels, and the complement of spiral ganglion neurons is similarly decreased, contributed to also by injury of the axons. The increase of protein in perilymph is reflected in the appearance of eosinophilic material within the scalae.

The effects of compression of brain tissue margining the cerebellopontine recess consist of the expected general features of degeneration, with rarefaction and gliosis, and with loss of neurons and demyelination of tracts. The cochlear nerve shows decrease in number of nerve fibers, those remaining presenting various degrees of degeneration of axis cylinders and myelin sheaths. Oligodendrocytes proliferate, and corpora amylacea increase in number (*see* Figures 68 A, B & C).

MENINGIOMA

Meningioma accounts for some 20 percent of intracranial neoplasms (Shambaugh, 1967a). This tumor type may arise in the cerebellopontine recess or rarely within the inner acoustic meatus, and it may produce the same pathophysiologic effects as neurofibroma. It may occur along with neurofibroma, especially in von Recklinghausen's disease (Nager, 1964b). Point of origin may be the surface of the petrous bone. Meningioma (Nager, 1964a), although essentially a benign tumor (excluding sarcoma), and rarely if ever metastasizing (same exclusion), nevertheless has a capacity for invading cranial bone. In the case of the pyramid this may produce labyrinthine involvement over and above the aforementioned consequences of cerebellopontine or cochlear nerve alterations. The involved osseous tissue, at the same time, tends to react with the hyperplastic production of new bone.

The gross positional features of meningioma affecting the

Figure 66A. Small, asymptomatic neurofibroma shown *in situ* arising from vestibular nerve. There is no degeneration of cochlear neurons. Illustration courtesy Schuknecht, *Pathology of the Ear,* Harvard University Press, 1974. Figure 66B. An unusual tumor equivalent of acoustic neurofibroma, composed of bundles of connective tissue fibers and appearing to arise from the split and widened lamina cribrosa (membrana perforata), seen arching over the upper margin of the tumor. Histologic section courtesy Dr. George Kelemen.

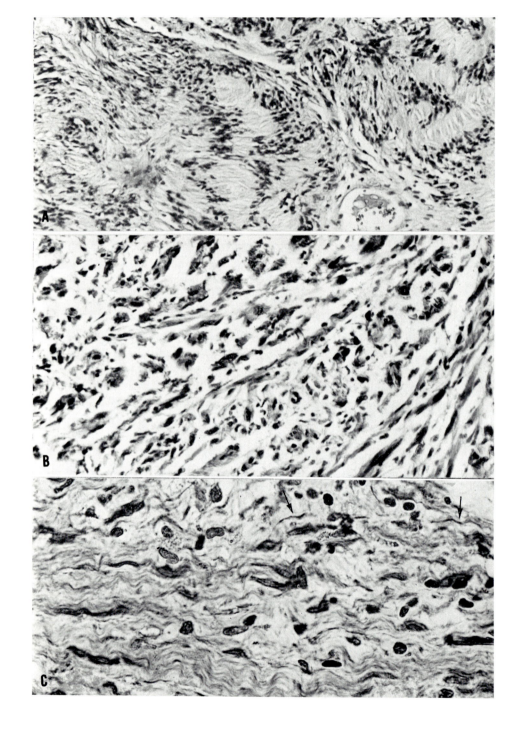

auditory tissues are the same as in neurofibroma. The tumor tends to be ovoid, less often flat and plaque-like.

Microscopically, meningioma is of two cellular types, understandably representing the basic active components of the pia-arachnoid. Mesothelioma is made up of arachnoidal villi growing in a whorled pattern, the cells sometimes being arranged more diffusely in sheets. Focal impregnation with calcium and/or iron produces psammoma bodies. Fibroma is composed of the fusiform leptomeningeal fibrocytes; it does not differ from fibroma of other situations. The two cellular components may appear together.

EPIDERMOID CYST

This is essentially a congenital malformation originating from embryonic rest. It is the third tumor type that may arise in the cerebellopontine recess with appreciable frequence; corresponding symptoms are produced. Age centers around twenty-five to forty years with male preponderance. Rupture may produce meningitis. Malignant forms do not appear (*see* Figures 69 A & B).

Grossly, the cyst may be rounded, or may be lobulated as a result of multilocular structure. The content is white and flaking, representing its keratinic nature. Microscopically, the wall of the cyst or of its locules is thin and fibrous, covered internally by stratified squamous epithelium desquamating keratinized epithelial cells into the cyst lumen. This material tends to degenerate; owing to a substantial lipoid content of the degenerated cells, cholesterol is liberated, together with other fatty material, resulting in the unsatisfactory term cholesteatoma.

← ————————————————————⧼⧼⧼

Figure 67. Acoustic neurofibroma, histologic patterns.
Figure 67A. Tumor consisting mainly of Schwann cells in characteristic palisades.
Figure 67B. Tumor is composed of fully-formed nerve fibers.
Figure 67C. Field showing Schwann cells as main component, Bodian stain. Short segments of axons are seen (arrows indicate examples).

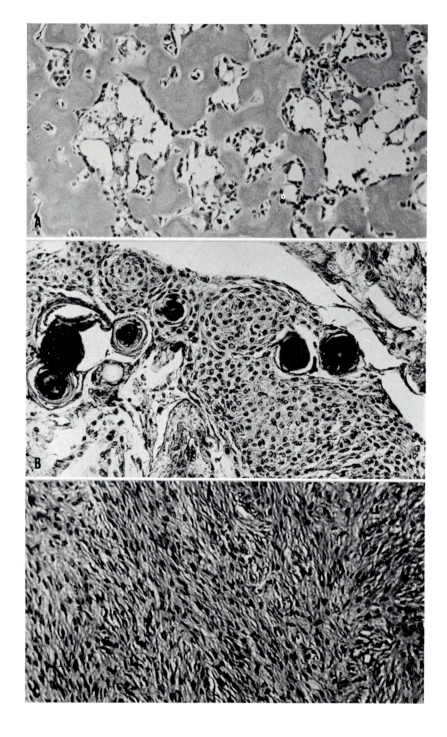

TERATOMA

Teratoma has been reported occurring in the internal auditory meatus in a case of trisomy 13-15. Striated muscle and nerve fibers were observed (Maniglia, Wolff and Herques, 1970).

LEUKEMIA, LYMPHOMA AND RELATED NEOPLASTIC PROCESSES

Leukemia affects the labyrinth mainly by hemorrhage. The cochlear nerve maybe infiltrated (Igarashi, 1972; Paparella, Berlinger, Oda *et al.,* 1972; Schuknecht, 1974). Lymphoma may involve the cochlear nerve and modiolus. Free cells may occasionally be found in the scalae (Paparella and El Fiky, 1972; Sando, Black, Randolph *et al.,* 1969). Myeloma may involve the temporal bone, but this usually is overshadowed by the manifestations of systemic disease (Schuknecht, 1974) (*see* Figures 70 A & B).

RETICULOSES

Histiocytosis-X is reported involving the temporal bone (Cohn, Sataloff and Lindsay, 1970; Lopez-Rios, Benitez and Vivar, 1969; Perlman, 1973). Hearing loss is primarily conductive; in cases of relatively extensive involvement the endocochlear tissues are affected, producing sensorineural hearing loss.

GLOMUS JUGULARE TUMOR

Glomus tissue is found in the adventitia of the dome of the jugular bulb (Guild, 1941) and along the course of the tympanic branch of the glossopharyngeal nerve and the auricular branch of

←————————————————————◀︎

Figure 68. Meningioma.
Figure 68A. Osteoid bone is formed by petrous pyramid in response to tumor.
Histologic types of meningioma:
Figure 68B. Mesothelioma, originating from arachnoidal villi.
Figure 68C. Fibroma.
Figure 68B, C from Dublin, Fundamentals of Neuropathology. Ed. II, Charles C Thomas, 1967.

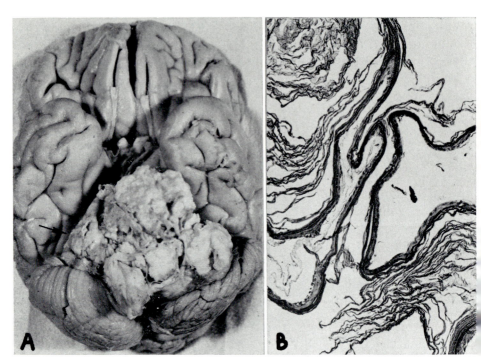

Figure 69. A. Epidermal cyst arising in the general region of the cerebello-pontine recess with extensive destruction of contiguous tissues. The remaining portion of pons is markedly degenerated (arrow). B. The cyst locules are lined by squamous epithelium, desquamating keratinized cells.

Illustration from Dublin, *Fundamentals of Neuropathology,* Ed. II, Charles C Thomas, 1967.

the vagus (Mawson, 1963). Tumors of this tissue tend first to invade the middle ear cavity, causing conductive deafness, but with more extensive involvement, sensorineural hearing loss may occur. The tumors are quite vascular and may bleed profusely. Histologically, they appear as lobulated masses of epithelial-like round to polyhedral cells with clear or acidophilic granular cytoplasm, surrounded by septa of highly vascular stroma. The tumor has an invasive capacity; distant metastases are uncommon. Over and above cochlear nerve disability, any cranial nerve from V to XII may be involved (Schuknecht, 1974). Glomus jugulare tumor is

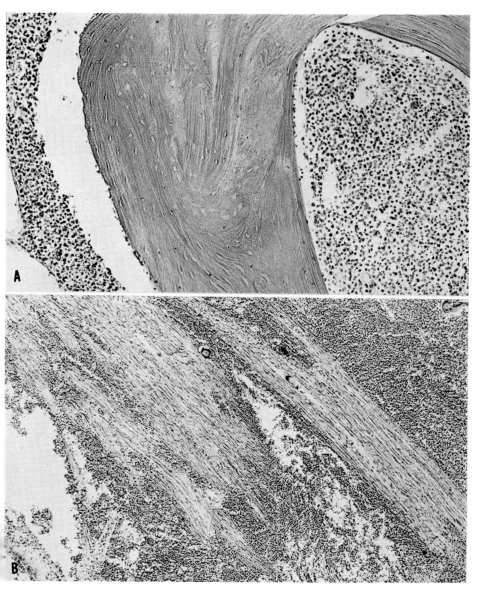

Figure 70. Leukemia.
Figure 70A. Infiltration of marrow spaces of petrous bone by immature lymphocytes.
Figure 70B. Same case. Hemorrhage into and around cochlear nerve.

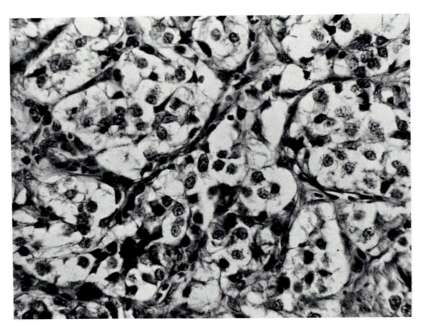

Figure 71. Glomus jugulare tumor. Round to ovoid tumor cells are even in structure, showing round to slightly ovoid stippled nuclei and clear, variably granular cytoplasm. The cells are arranged in ball-like clusters surrounded by connective tissue septa. The stroma is quite vascular.

regarded as nonchromaffin paraganglioma (Shambaugh, 1967a; Taylor, 1958). Norepinephrine secretion has been found in some cases (Balogh, Draskoczy and Caulfield, 1966; Duke, Boshell, Soteres *et al.,* 1964).

METASTATIC TUMORS

Metastatic involvement of the cochlea doubtless occurs more frequently than reported, but is overshadowed by the overall state of the malignant disease (Schuknecht, Allam and Murakami, 1968; Schuknecht, 1974). Sources include especially breast, kidney, lung, stomach, prostate and thyroid (Adams, Paparella and El Fiky, 1971).

Chapter 8

METABOLIC DISORDERS

THIS IS A RATHER UNSATISFACTORY categorical term inasmuch as most diseases involve abnormal metabolism; however, there are some disorders that appear essential and intrinsic, and not the result of evident processes such as congenital maldevelopment, infection, injury or neoplasia. Metabolic disorders could in substantial measure be classed as being of unknown cause, and a categorical group could be assembled under a heading of idiopathic; however, this feature could pertain as well to some disorders discussed previously as, for example, various tumors whose causes remain to be discovered. Neoplasms, nevertheless, have categorical character of new growth.

THE AGING PROCESS—PRESBYCUSIS

Senescence is a winding down of the time of human activity—a catabolic process engaged in by all who survive long enough, and deserving regard as a normal experience. Since aging, however, results in variable incapacity and ultimately in death, and, of import to the present discussion, in loss of hearing, this catabolic process will be treated as a disease.

Auditory disability consequent to aging is termed *presbycusis* (Bredberg, 1968; Engström, Ades and Andersson, 1966; Engström, Ades and Bredberg, 1970; Gacek and Schuknecht, 1969; Igarashi, 1972; Johnsson and Hawkins, 1972b; Schuknecht, 1974). The audiometric findings resemble those of acoustic overstimulation, and the question arises as to whether presbycusis is the result of cumulative exposure to sound (Engström, Ades and Andersson, 1966; Lebo and Redell, 1972); indeed, stresses are placed on the auditory system by various pathogenic factors throughout life (Schuknecht, 1974), some of them, as in the case of administration

173

of antibiotics, possibly lost from the case history.

The senescent changes of the auditory pathway are manifestations of a generalized process affecting tissues throughout the body. The interaction of organ systems prevails; the effects of diminished endocrine and alimentary function, for example, on neural tissues may be added to those intrinsic to aging per se.

Hearing deficits associated with aging tend characteristically to be sensorineural in the main (Gacek and Schuknecht, 1969). Clinicopathologic forms of presbycusis have been categorized on a basis of preponderant involvement of stria vascularis, organ of Corti, basilar membrane, spiral ganglion, or central pathway structures (Schuknecht, 1974); however, the categories are seldom observed singly, but tend, rather, to occur in combined form (Johnsson and Hawkins, 1972b). It would appear preferable to consider that they represent variations in the manifestation of a single disease process. Worthy of note, nevertheless, is the difference between symptoms of peripheral and central involvement. The percentile level of neuronal population required for effective integration of auditory impulses is greater than that for the perception of pure tones. The resulting loss of speech discrimination out of proportion to hearing loss for pure tones is termed *phonemic regression* (Gaeth, 1948).

Presbycusis illustrates well the need for including the pathologic study of the central part of the auditory pathway with that of the peripheral portion and for the inclusion of the state of the cochlear nuclei in the combined correlative audiogram.

With the aforementioned potentially-complicating factors of sound and antibiotics in the development of presbycusis, anoxia must now be included, as it is a frequently-encountered, basic pathogenic mechanism producing high-tone sensorineural hearing loss through cochlear nuclear injury, and most significantly, without apparent cochlear damage. Anoxia may be produced in a number of ways; as in the other aforementioned pathogenic factors, the incidents of its occurrence may not have been appreciated, or may have been forgotten.

The pathologic lesions of the auditory pathway in presbycusis (Bredberg, 1968; Johnsson and Hawkins, 1972a,b,c; Schuknecht,

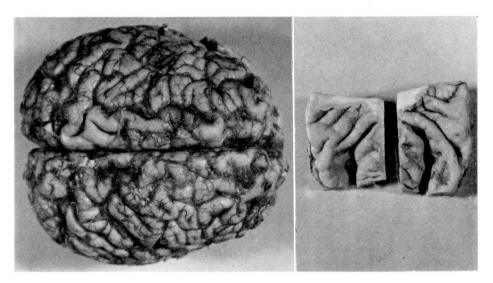

Figure 72. Gross photographs of brain from a case of presbycusis (man, aged 76). The cerebral vertex on the left and the two auditory areas on the right show convolutional atrophy.

1955, 1964) are, above all, variable in severity and distribution; this, rather than true disagreement, is the basis of differences among accounts by different workers. A didactic description of the stated lesions must properly remain in the nature of a presentation of general principles.

The state of the blood vascular supply is pertinent. The degeneration of organ of Corti and spiral ganglion observed in presbycusis may be caused, at least in a measure, by microangiopathy (Johnsson and Hawkins, 1972b). The development of arteriosclerosis in tissues throughout the body tends to increase with age to an extent where it is a moot point, whether vascular sclerosis should be regarded as an independent process or simply as a part of senescence. It is certain that there is a gradual involution of vessels of the membranous wall of the cochlea and of the system of spiral vessels of the basilar membrane and vestibular lip, with hyaline thickening of some arterioles that remain present. The elements of the cochlear duct are involved with angiosclerosis and atrophy,

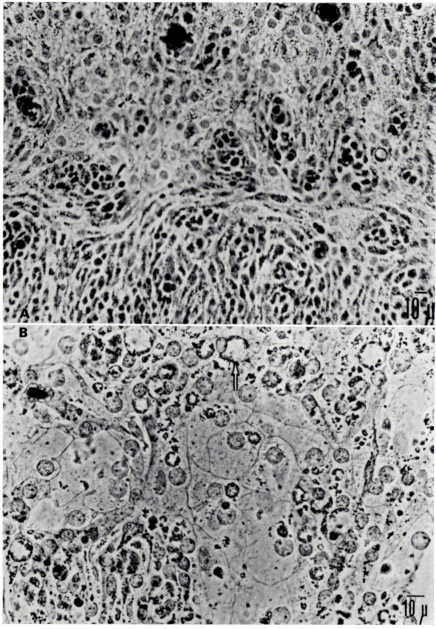

Figure 73. Changes of maturation and of aging in vestibular membrane.
Figure 73A. Surface preparation of membrane from woman aged sixteen,
presumably normal. Compare with Figure 5.

especially of the stria vascularis, found notably in the lower half of the basal turn (Saxen, 1952). Surface preparations show the process well. Thickened capillary walls tend to be PAS-positive (Jörgensen, 1964). Comparison may be made with retinal vascular changes.

In man, sensorineural degeneration with aging has been found invariably associated with some degree of atrophy of the stria vascularis. The latter process (Johnsson and Hawkins, 1972a; Schuknecht, Watanuki, Takahashi *et al.*, 1974) may produce hearing loss, possibly through failure to maintain the normal ionic balance of endolymph, and this may lead in time to degeneration of hair cells. The atrophic stria vascularis, especially the epithelium, appears thinner than usual (Saxen, 1952). There may be incorporation of pigment.

In presbycusis the epithelial cells covering the inferior surface of the vestibular membrane appear vacuolated (Johnsson, 1971). With advancing age this epithelial layer exhibits a process of disorganization that appears to be an extension of the normal process of maturation.

Atrophy of elements of the organ of Corti is noteworthy. The outer hair cells are prone to degenerate early, more so than inner hair cells, and especially toward the base of the cochlea (Johnsson and Hawkins, 1972b; Schuknecht, 1974). The organ of Corti appears more or less lowered and deformed; exclusion of artifact is requisite (Saxen, 1952). The sensory cell changes are roughly paralleled by alterations in nonsensory or supporting elements, especially if inner hair cells are injured.

The most nearly constant finding in the cochlea in old age has been found to consist of atrophy of the spiral ganglion and of the nerves in the osseous spiral lamina; these changes are evident especially in the lower basal turn, tending to spread upward with increasing age (Bredberg, 1968). Loss of nerve cells and fibers appears related particularly to that of inner hair cells; however, since the outer hair cells are supplied by a scant minority of afferent

Figure 73B. Same, from woman aged sixty-eight. In addition to irregularity of shape and enlargement of cells, large vacuoles appear (arrow indicates one). Illustrations courtesy Johnson, *Ann Otol, 80:*425, 1971.

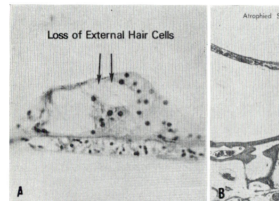

Loss of External Hair Cells

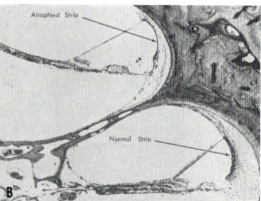

Atrophied Stria

Normal Stria

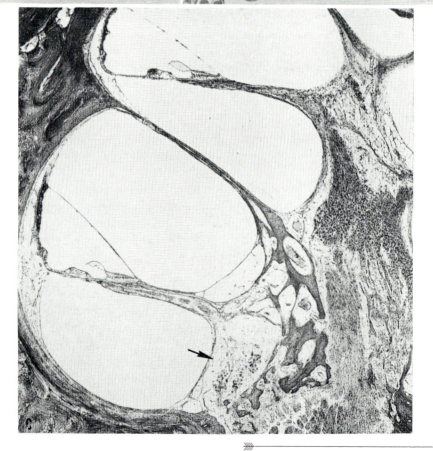

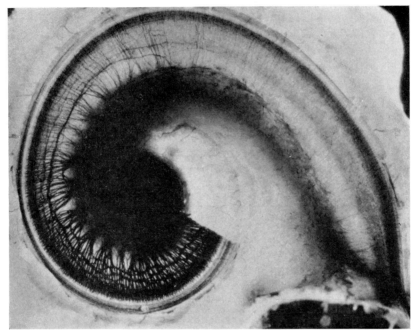

Figure 75. Presbycusis, man aged seventy-three. Whole surface mount, basal coil, prepared with nerve stain. There is almost complete degeneration of nerve fibers and organ of Corti in the lower portion of the coil. Illustration courtesy of Bredberg, *Acta Otolaryngol,* Suppl. 236, 1968.

fibers (Spoendlin, 1971), loss of these few bundles might escape notice, while degeneration of the relatively numerous radial fibers to inner hair cells will be more evident.

Changes of age affecting the central portion of the auditory pathway represent an important division of neuropathology. This includes especially senile and presenile dementia, involving deterioration of intellect, with commensurate objective elusiveness of

Figure 74. Presbycusis.
Figure 74A. Loss of external hair cells. After Schuknecht, *Pathology of the Ear,* Harvard University Press, 1974.
Figure 74B. Atrophy of the stria vascularis. After Schuknecht *et al; Laryngoscope, 84*:1777, 1974.
Figure 74C. Same case as Figure 72. Reduction of neurons of spiral ganglion in basal turn (arrow).

the state of hearing. Simple, general changes of senescence without such specific intellectual deterioration provide more of an opportunity for auditory evaluation. Few specific, well-controlled central auditory pathway studies have been reported. Involution of the different centers has been surveyed; to date such studies have not been based on a proper appreciation of cellular architecture.

Opinion varies as to location of maximal injury; the superior temporal gyrus has been found most severely involved among cortical regions (Brody, 1955). Atrophy and degeneration of ganglion cells was found throughout the central auditory pathway, resulting in elevation of auditory threshold essentially for high frequencies, together with impairment of speech discrimination and binaural synthesis. In some cases, impairment of speech discrimination was found in the presence of almost normal pure-tone thresholds. The pathologic changes were uniform in the ventral cochlear nucleus and medial geniculate body, with various degrees of degeneration of the dorsal olivary complex and inferior colliculus (Kirikae, Sato and Shitara, 1964). A reduction in numbers of cells was encountered together with pigment, the latter especially in the ventral cochlear nucleus. High-tone hearing loss was attributed to the original availability of a smaller number of nerve fibers for higher frequencies.

The cellular changes observed in senescence (Andrew, 1956) consist of shrinkage of cells, with increase of pericellular spaces; cell outlines may be irregular. Various stages of nuclear dissolution may appear. Nissl substance may be decreased or lost. Lipofuscin may appear. Especially in the frontal cortex and hippocampus, senile plaques and Alzheimer's neurofibrillary change may be observed, especially in cases of dementia (Dublin, 1967).

Variability of involvement of the central auditory structures is noteworthy; such variation is individually intrinsic in basis, and the mechanism is not understood. The findings in an unselected case are demonstrated in the accompanying illustrations. Of special interest in the ventral cochlear nucleus is a tendency toward high-frequency or dorsal zonal involvement. Spheroid cells are notably involved. Reparative gliosis is marked. In the inferior colliculus, aside from basic loss of neuronal elements, nerve cell deterioration

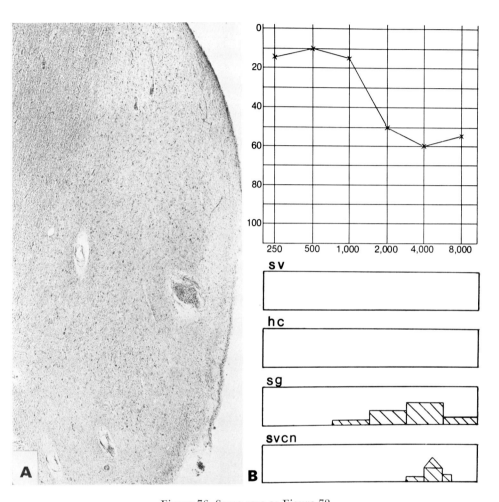

Figure 76. Same case as Figure 72.

Figure 76A. Transverse section through superior ventral cochlear nucleus for general orientation (see Fig. 77).

Figure 76B. Combined correlated audiogram showing audiometric curve and estimate of injury of component elements. (sv) Stria vascularis. (nc) Hair cells. (cn) Cochlear neurons. (svcn) Spheroid cells of superior ventral cochlear nucleus, injury estimated at ventrodorsally progressive levels of the nucleus corresponding to frequency levels of the audiogram with low frequencies ventral and high frequencies dorsal (see Fig. 41). This element must be included in any combined correlated audiographic chart.

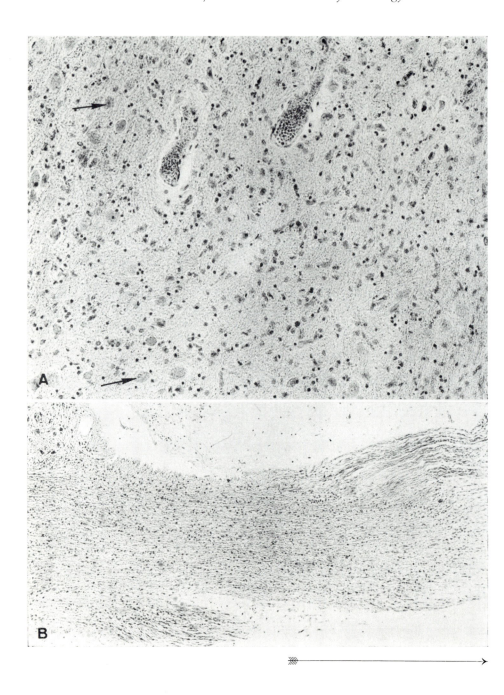

and increase of glia disrupt the laminated pattern and impart a somewhat rough character to the histologic pattern. Cell degeneration, with diminution of nerve cell population, and with disturbance of laminated pattern, is seen also, variably, in medical geniculate body and auditory cortex (*see* Figures 76-81) .

HYPERTENSION AND ARTERIOSCLEROSIS

Some features of vascular sclerosis were presented in the discussion of presbycusis.

Hypertensive vascular disease is regarded as a basis for sudden hearing loss, possibly through a mechanism of vasoconstriction (Polus, 1972) , the auditory pathway sharing such effects with the remainder of the central nervous system. Psychomotor features require consideration. Unfortunately, the cochlear vessels are not amenable to direct clinical observation as are retinal vessels, but the condition appears comparable. Atheromatous microembolism also may occur.

In one report no correlation was found between hypertension and perceptive hearing impairment (Hansen, 1968b) ; in the same group a correlation was found between impairment of hearing and brain degeneration, apparently arteriosclerotic.

Occlusion of terminal branches of the labyrinthine arterial tree should inevitably have clinical manifestations as encountered in otologic practice. Hearing losses of varying segments as to frequency can result from lesions of segmental cochlear arterioles. Patchy degenerative changes in organ of Corti and stria vascularis

Figure 77A. Higher power view of a field of the upper portion of Figure 76A. The two venules in upper midcenter serve for orientation. Injury of spheroid cells is less clear than in Figure 42 since in the present case the process is not in active progress; also, the spheroid cells in the present case are obscured somewhat by gliosis. They are reduced in number, a few ghost residuals being seen, in a triangular zone with base to right and apex to left, extending across the middle portion of the field; the relatively well-preserved spheroid cells that remain are reduced in number; they are concentrated especially along the upper and lower margins of the field, especially in the upper and lower left-hand corners (arrows indicate two such cells).

Figure 77B. Central or glial portion of cochlear nerve shows atrophy and gliosis. See also Figure 74C.

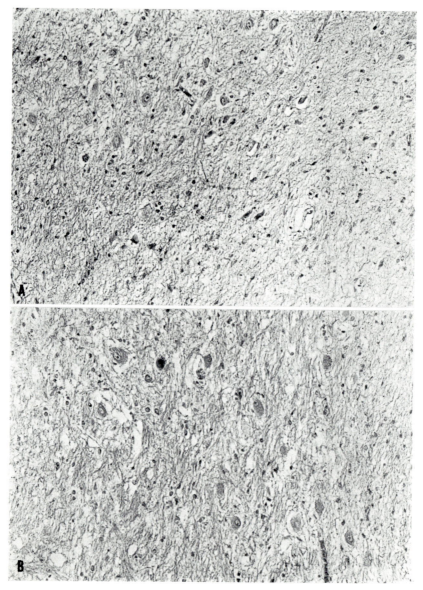

Figure 78. Presbycusis, woman aged one hundred and two. Upper (Figure 78A) and lower (Figure 78B) portions of superior ventral cochlear nucleus show loss of spheroid cells with general tissue rarefaction throughout the nucleus, more severe in the upper portion.

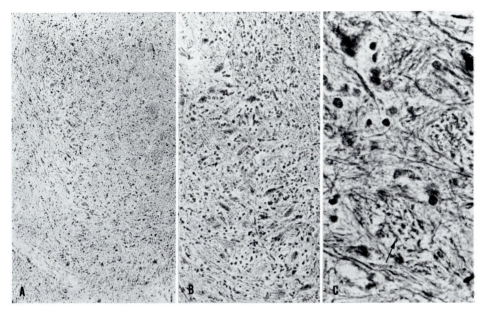

Figure 79. Presbycusis involving medial dorsal cochlear nucleus.
Figure 79A. Same case as in Figure 76 showing severe loss of neurons, with gliosis, the medial dorsal olivary nucleus extending in a band from upper left to lower right.
Figure 79B. Presbycusis (another case) showing varying injury of the fusiform nerve cells with reduction in number. There is intense reactive gliosis.
Figure 79C. Higher power of Figure 79B. Bodian stain, showing degeneration and reduction in number of cells and nerve fibers. In the circular clusters of fibers seen in cross section (arrow indicates one such cluster) the granular material represents yellow pigment, apparently lipochrome ("wear-and-tear" effect).

have been produced with experimental vascular occlusion and point to a segmentally-arranged blood supply within the peripheral cochlear system (Alford, Shaver, Rosenberg *et al.,* 1965). Effects of experimental compromise of the main arterial and venous circulation to the cochlea were presented previously (Kimura and Perlman, 1956, 1958). The cochlea tends to be involved as a whole; maximal injury may be apical. In subarachnoid hemorrhage of hypertensive (or other) origin, blood may pass through the

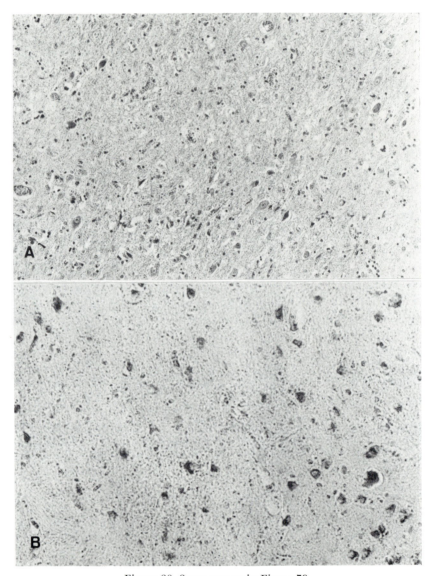

Figure 80. Same case as in Figure 79.

Figure 80A. Central nucleus of inferior colliculus. There is loss of nerve cells with general tissue rarefaction and gliosis and with general disorganization of tissue pattern. Compare with Figure 31C.

Figure 80B. Ventral nucleus of medial geniculate body showing some degree of loss of nerve cells with slight gliosis and tissue rarefaction. Compare with Figure 34B.

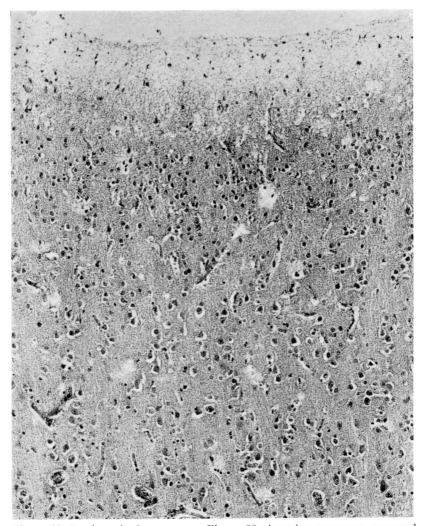

Figure 81. Presbycusis. Same case as Figure 80. Anterior transverse temporal convolution showing narrowing of the cortex with irregular loss of nerve cells and disorganization of the columnated pattern. Compare with Figure 37B.

cochlear aqueduct, especially when the latter is larger than average. There may be passage also through the modiolus into the perilymphatic scalae (Holden and Schuknecht, 1968) (*see* Figures 82-83).

The central portion of the auditory pathway may be similarly

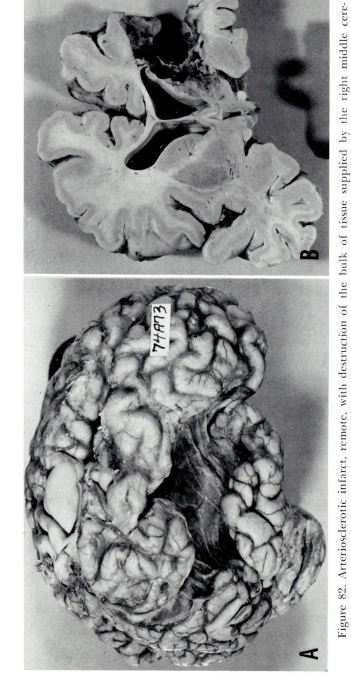

Figure 82. Arteriosclerotic infarct, remote, with destruction of the bulk of tissue supplied by the right middle cerebral artery. Figure 82A, supralateral surface view; Figure 82B, transverse section. The auditory cortex and radiation are included in the tissue destroyed. See also Figure 32A (same case).

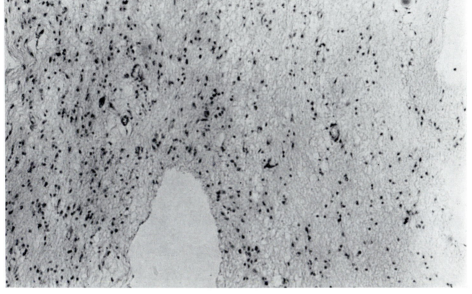

Figure 83 .Same case as in Figure 82. Ventral division of right medial geniculate body with pial surface to right. There is replacement of the normal tissue by a glial web.

involved in arterial insufficiency. The cochlear nuclear complex is involved in anterior inferior cerebellar occlusion (Adams, 1943). (Necrosis of the membranous labyrinth also may result [Schuknecht, 1974]) . The more central portions of the auditory pathway may be similarly affected, tending, however, to be a part of infarction of a severely incapacitating nature in the case of brain stem involvement wherein the state of hearing may be relatively unimportant or difficult to evaluate, and in cases of unilateral temporal lobe infarction the effect on hearing will be inconstant.

A correlation was found between hearing loss and degree of arteriosclerosis. Adventitial hyaline thickening was observed of the arteries of the internal auditory meatus in relation to age (Fisch, Dobozi and Greig, 1972) . A correlation has been reported between hypercholesterolemia and hearing loss with implication of arteriosclerosis as a pathogenic factor (Rosen and Rosen, 1971; Spencer, 1973) .

Injury of the nervous system owing to hypertension and arterio-sclerosis accounts for a considerable segment of neuropathology. Specific auditory pathway studies have been few and are needed.

ANOXIA

A ready supply of oxygen is essential to the adequate function of the organ of Corti. This need appears to be met by the vascular network beneath the hearing organ. In anoxia, glucose level in the organ of Corti and perilymph declines, as does also the essential adenosine triphosphatase of the organ of Corti and stria vascularis (Spector and Lucente, 1974; Thalman, Miyoshi and Thalman, 1972). Endolymph sodium rises and potassium falls; the change is greater than that resulting from stimulation with excessive sound (Suga, Preston and Snow, 1970).

Among the special senses, however, hearing is not the most vul-nerable to anoxia; it is not affected by oxygen want corresponding to as high as 40,000 feet altitude, and is maintained when vision has failed (Wever, Lawrence, Hemphill *et al.*, 1949). In experimental animals extremes of anoxia necessary to produce deterioration of potentials (Spector and Lucente, 1974) has resulted in damage to the heart, causing death (Lawrence and Wever, 1952).

Anoxia as a pathogenic mechanism may result from a number of initial causes. It appears to be the prime factor in kernicterus (Dublin, 1949); essentially the same pathogenesis and pathologic alterations are encountered in neonatal asphyxia, which may be followed by cerebral palsy, attended in some cases by hearing loss. The audiometric features of postanoxic hearing defect resemble those of the high-tone hearing loss produced by hemolytic disease (Fisch, 1955). Hearing is affected in various other anoxic condi-tions such as post-carbon monoxide asphyxial state. Oxygen want is to be numbered among those incidents of living that may be com-bined in a cumulative insult to the auditory system, and often un-suspected or forgotten.

The gradient of involvement of the portions of the auditory pathway in anoxia highlights the need for including the central portion in pathologic studies of the auditory pathway.

The organ of Corti and spiral ganglion show no appreciable

histologic alteration consequent to anoxia (Buch, Tygstrup and Jörgensen, 1966; Dublin, 1974; Gerrard, 1952). Experimental results (guinea pigs and cats) are confirmatory (Falbe-Hansen, Christensen, Gesselson *et al.,* 1958).

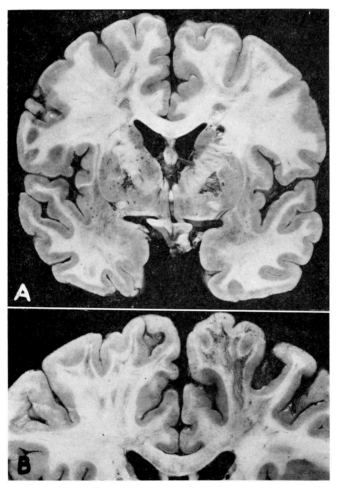

Figure 84. Gross photographs of severe post-anoxic encephalopathy.
Figure 84A. Bilateral degeneration of globus pallidus is seen.
Figure 84B. Shows degeneration of subcortical white matter. Illustration from Dublin, *Fundamentals of Neuropathology,* Ed. II, Charles C Thomas, 1967.

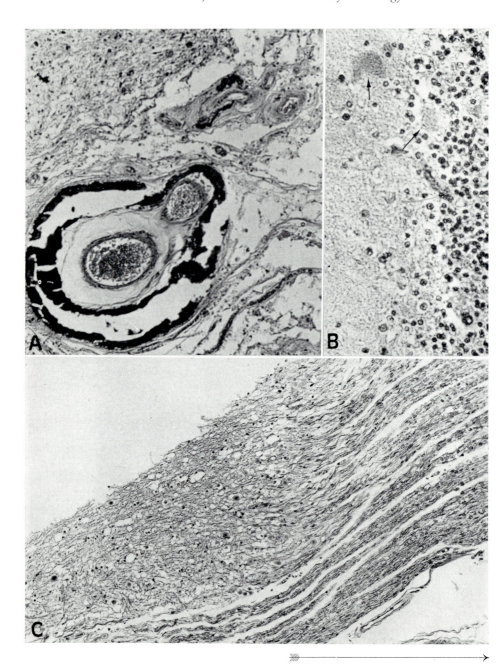

The postanoxic alterations of the central nervous system form one of the notable segments of neuropathology. There is a topistic gradient of vulnerability. Heavily involved centers include especially the lenticular nucleus, notably the globus pallidus, athetosis being a noteworthy clinical residual; the latter center may cavitate, and arteries and nerve cells may show encrustation with iron and/ or calcium. Hippocampus and dentate nucleus also are susceptible. Regions of cortex and subcortical white matter are variably degenerated. The auditory pathway centers may be affected along with, but not necessarily more severely than, the brain generally (Buch, Tygstrup and Jörgensen, 1966). (Hearing loss in athetoids, especially for high frequencies, is well-recognized [Flottorp, Morley and Skatvedt, 1957].) The features outlined previously in relation to the cochlear nuclei in kernicterus apply similarly to anoxia per se. There is a gradient of severity of involvement of the ventral cochlear nucleus, especially of the superior division, the dorsal portion of the nucleus being affected more severely than the ventral. This is in keeping with the high-frequency-dorsal to low-frequency-ventral tonotopic architecture of the ventral cochlear nucleus and the high-tone character of the hearing loss. The spheroid cells are notably involved. In cases of remote onset, reactive gliosis is observed. The dorsal cochlear nucleus is not affected appreciably by anoxia; its alteration plays no significant part in postanoxic deafness. This is in keeping with the regressive character of the dorsal cochlear nucleus.

The inferior colliculi are involved in anoxia. In experimental asphyxia neonatorum of the monkey the central nucleus may be destroyed while the cortex is spared (Ranck and Windle, 1959). It was shown in a much earlier investigation that only deep lesions of the inferior colliculi produced gross hearing defects in animals (von Bechterew, 1895, quoted by Geniec and Morest, 1971). The

Figure 85. Carbon monoxide anoxia, remote.
Figure 85A. Globus pallidus. Cystic degeneration is seen, with mineral encrustation of small arteries.
Figure 85B. Cerebellum, showing loss of Purkinje cells; two degenerated remnants are seen at top (arrows).
Figure 85C. Degeneration of cochlear nerve.

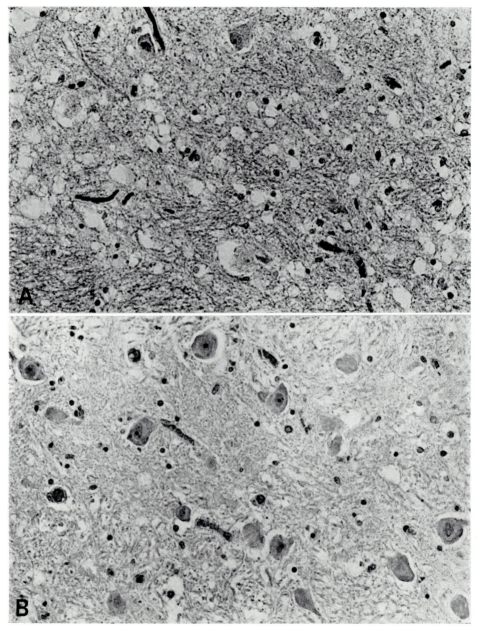

Figure 86. Same case as in Figure 85. Superior ventral cochlear nucleus showing severe loss of spheroid cells in upper zone (86A) and more moderate cell loss in lower zone (86B).

medial geniculate bodies also may be involved. Auditory cortex and subcortical white matter are affected variably. The extra-auditory cortical alterations may result in intellectual deterioration.

SICKLE CELL DISEASE

Sickling results in microcirculatory obstruction, with involvement of the stria vascularis, and with degeneration of the structures of the cochlear duct (Morgenstein and Manace, 1969).

ENDOCRINE DISORDERS

Diabetes

Auditory dysfunction is observed in about 50 percent of diabetics. PAS-positive thickening of capillary walls in stria vascularis is typical but not specific (Igarashi, 1972). The alteration is similar to that in arteriosclerosis, but tends to be more severe; there appears to be a correlation with various diabetic complications without necessary relation to age (Jörgensen, 1964). The increased general severity of arteriosclerosis in diabetics affects the state of central nervous system tissues. The structures of the auditory pathway share in such involvement, but not specifically or notably. Neuronal degeneration has been observed especially in the basal turn of the cochlea, in keeping with high frequency hearing loss (Schuknecht, 1974). Involvement of the cochlear nerve or nucleus comparable with that of the optic nerve, attributable to diabetes per se, has not been observed.

Experimental insulin hypoglycemia leads to a decrease in endolymph potassium and a rise of sodium. The high potassium/sodium ratio appears maintained by a process ultimately utilizing glucose as source of energy (Mendelsohn and Roderique, 1972).

Thyroid Dysfunction

Hypothyroidism is considered to cause clinically detectable functional changes within the inner ear. Cases have been reported of perceptive deafness, with improvement on administration of thyroid substance (Lawrence, 1960). Definitive studies appear needed (Schuknecht, 1974). Confirmatory pathologic studies are not available (Igarashi, 1972). Hypothyroidism is considered to play a part in the pathogenesis of Meniere's syndrome.

NUTRITIONAL DEFICIENCY

Auditory dysfunction has been observed in experimental avitaminosis (Igarashi, 1972). Segmental demyelination of cochlear nerves, with hearing loss, has been reported in malnutrition and cachexia (Gussen, 1974). The problem requires further study.

SYSTEMIC DISORDERS OF LIPOID METABOLISM

The widespread intraneuronal accumulation of lipoid material in amaurotic family idiocy illustrates the involvement in varying degrees of the structures of the auditory pathway in processes affecting the nervous system as a whole. On such a basis auditory pathology could consist of an account of neural histopathology in its entirety. The scope of the present discussion, however, is determined by auditory pathway lesions resulting in clinically manifest and objectively documented disorders of hearing, standing out in that special and individual way among the clinical findings.

LABYRINTHINE OSTEOPOROSIS

In the past this condition has been known as otosclerosis (Altmann, 1962; Engström and Röckert, 1962; Igarashi, 1972; Lindsay, 1973b,c; Nager, 1969b; Schuknecht, 1974; Shambaugh, 1967a), a term that is unsatisfactory in that it refers to the ear rather than to the osseous labyrinth, within whose confines the disorder is found almost exclusively, and in that it does not denote the basic pathologic process. To date the disorder has appeared only in the human. Incidence is generally stated to be higher in females, although some reservation has been voiced (Larsson, 1962). Heredity appears to be a factor, although the mode of inheritance is not established (Larsson, 1962). Histologic alteration resembling labyrinthine osteoporosis has been reported in human subjects following deep irradiation of the head (Jörgensen and Kristensen, 1966) and in dogs receiving cobalt irradiation (Mendoza, Rius, de Stefani *et al.*, 1969). In a case of deep irradiation to the head the

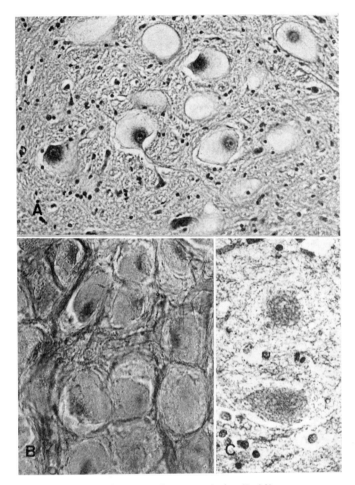

Figure 87. Cases of amaurotic family idiocy.

Figure 87A. Anterior horn cells are distended with lipoid substance. Illustration from Dublin, *Fundamentals of Neuropathology,* Ed. II, Charles C Thomas, 1967.

Figure 87B. Same condition, another case, involving the spiral ganglion. Illustration courtesy Dr. George Kelemen.

Figure 87C. Batten type of amaurotic family idiocy. Two spheroid cells of superior ventral cochlear nucleus show lipoid material stained in a positive way with luxol fast blue (photographed with yellow filter), the cell membranes and processes being less well-visualized. Histologic section courtesy Dr. Mary M. Herman.

author found hyaline sclerosis of blood vessels but nothing suggesting osteoporosis. Coincidental occurrence of osteoporosis must be considered in such a case.

The cause of labyrinthine osteoporosis is unknown. The basic pathologic process consists of the resorption of bone, with the formation of spaces in which mesenchymal cells and loose connective tissue appear. Blood vessels are dilated. In due course the spaces are filled with more compact fibrous tissue. The bone exhibits a sieve-like pattern. In a later, relatively inactive stage the spongy bone may be calcified, less vascular, and more solid. Some relatively large spaces may remain filled with fibrous and adipose tissue. The pathologic bone in labyrinthine osteoporosis tends to be basophilic. This, together with a certain pattern formation, has resulted in the term blue mantles. This terminology is of no practical import and does not merit further consideration.

The osteoporotic process tends to arise in relation to the cartilaginous tissue of the endochondral layer; a frequent but not exclusive point of origin is the fissula ante fenestram. The virtual confinement of the disorder to the osseous labyrinthine capsule appears to be related to the individual character of that structure.

The most common complication affecting auditory function is fixation of the stapes. Of importance to the present discussion, sensorineural hearing loss appears in some cases (Linthicum, 1966; Ruedi, 1962; Shambaugh, 1973), most often down-sloping high frequency in type, with good speech discrimination, and with recruitment in most instances. In cases showing such manifestations, labyrinthine osteoporosis should be considered in the diagnosis (Carhart, 1966).

The basis of the hearing loss is not fully understood and is the subject of debate. Cochlear involvement in the dysplastic process may be manifest and may result in distortion of the capsular and modiolar architecture. In such cases the stria vascularis may be disorganized, and there may be some loss of hair cells and spiral ganglion neurons. Nonosteoporotic bone may be formed within the scalae in relation to overlying osteoporotic foci, with replacement of the endosteum. Especially the scala tympani may, on occasion, be filled completely with such newly-formed bone. Correlation of deafness with fibrous thickening of the endosteum, especially underlying the stria vascularis, has been reported (Linthicum, 1972). Probably of great import is the extension of osteoporotic bone, in some cases, through endosteum into the labyrinthine channel. The soft structures of the cochlea, however, appear to be in better health in many cases than the audiogram would indicate, and the histologic status may not be adequate for establishing firmly the intravital correlates (Kelemen and Linthicum, 1969).

The absence of consistent pathologic findings has led to an effort to explain the sensorineural hearing loss in labyrinthine osteoporosis on a basis of biochemical alteration of the endocochlear fluid, induced by the encroaching dysplastic bone (Ruedi, 1962). Alkaline phosphatase has been found in perilymph (Lawrence, 1966b, Ruedi and Spoendlin, 1966). Significant correlation is reported of hydrolases in perilymph with the progress of sensorineural hearing loss; this is thought to point to labyrinthine osteoporosis as an enzymatic disorder, with disturbance of enzyme balance (Chevance, Causse, Bretlau *et al.*, 1972).

OSTEITIS DEFORMANS

In osteitis deformans (Clemis, Boyles, Harford *et al.*, 1967; Perlman, 1973; Schuknecht, 1974) the temporal bone may be involved; the osseous labyrinth is last to be affected, and then only in the most severe cases. The periosteal layer is involved first, and the endochondral and endosteal layers, later. Sensorineural hearing loss appears regularly, affecting especially high frequencies. Its pathologic basis is not evident except for those cases in which the dysplastic bone involves the sensory and neural cochlear components. The comparative paucity of pathologic material prevents optimal correlation of structural alterations with auditory disability. Since the hearing loss may be sensorineural, the central portion of the auditory pathway—notably, the cochlear nuclei—must be included in pathologic studies to provide whole auditory pathway-oriented findings.

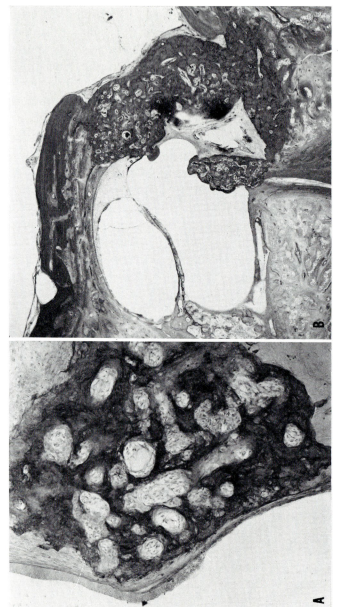

Figure 88. Labyrinthine osteoporosis with involvement of the perilymphatic spaces. Zones of endosteal fibrosis are seen. Figure 88A. The basic process of labyrinthine osteoporosis is illustrated with enlarged spaces occupied by mesenchymal tissue; the overall osseous pattern is sieve-like. Figure 88B. The pathologic bone protrudes into the scala tympani. Illustrations courtesy Dr. Fred H. Linthicum, Jr.

HYPEROSTOSIS OF THE FORAMINA OF THE OSSEOUS LAMINA CRIBOSA

The bundles of the cochlear nerve have been observed to be compromised as they traverse the foramina in the central base of the modiolus, by deposits of bone about the margins of the foramina. The alteration is reported to occur first in the region of the basal coil (Krmpotic-Nemanic, Nemanic and Kostovic, 1972).

MENIERE'S SYNDROME

This disorder (House, 1968; Igarashi, 1972; Pulec, 1968; Schuknecht, 1974; Shambaugh, 1967a) is manifested by episodic vertigo, tinnitus and fluctuating hearing loss. The latter more often is unilateral, but may be bilateral, and is of sensorineural type, affecting low frequencies especially but with flat audiometric curve in later stages. Loudness recruitment is characteristically present (Schuknecht, 1968b).

The basic pathophysiologic factor in Meniere's syndrome is increase of hydrostatic pressure within the cochlear duct in the presence of which the sensorineural elements cannot function effectively (McCabe and Ryu, 1968; Schuknecht, 1968b, 1974; Simmons, 1968). As an experimental correlate, on the injection into the cochlear duct (guinea pig) of a solution comparable with endolymph as to electrolyte content, with increase of pressure, the A-C potential response decreased commensurately and returned to baseline on release of pressure (McCabe and Wolsk, 1961). The disordered functional state appeared to be concerned with hydrostatic pressure rather than with chemical alteration.

An important pathologic condition predisposing to Meniere's-type episodes consists of inability of the endolymphatic sac to reabsorb endolymph or to compensate for pressure changes within the cochlear duct. Under such circumstances vascular overload in the stria vascularis, with increased capillary permeability, may precipitate a Meniere's-type attack. This may result in some cases from an allergic hypersensitivity reaction with liberation of histamine (Clemis, 1972; Powers, 1973; Pulec, 1972; Williams, 1968). Emotional stress also may play a part as in situational stress (Williamson and Gifford, 1971). Among the contributory medical conditions in Meniere's syndrome are hypothyroidism, adrenal-pituitary insufficiency and disordered glucose metabolism (Powers, 1972). Among the several disease processes that produce the clinical equivalent of Meniere's syndrome, congenital syphilis is noteworthy.

The final initiating event in a severe vertiginous attack is thought to be rupture of the vestibular membrane with intermingling of perilymph and endolymph, normally maintained at different electrolyte concentrations by the intact membranes (Igarashi, 1972; Lawrence and McCabe, 1959; McCabe and Ryu, 1968; Schuknecht, 1974; Simmons, 1968). Experimental rupture of the vestibular membrane, however, did not produce alteration of threshold for low frequencies (Schuknecht and El Seifi, 1963). A hypothesis contrary to the foregoing one is that the membrane rupture affords relief from an attack rather than initiating one. Patients have stated that they heard a snap in the ear at the moment of relief (House, 1968). The more one reflects on the pathogenesis of Meniere's syndrome, the more one suspects that it is a hydrodynamic rather than a biochemical disorder and, as such, is comparable to glaucoma.

On pathologic examination the outstanding feature within the cochlea is endolymphatic hydrops (Hallpike and Cairns, 1938). The vestibular membrane is displaced, and this may obliterate the scala vestibuli. This is more marked at the apex, where the vestibular membrane is thought to be less resistant to pressure changes than in the more basal turns. Evidence of rupture and healing, variably, of the vestibular membrane may be observed.

The endolymphatic sac appears avascular grossly, in vivo (Shambaugh, 1969). Microscopically there is subepithelial fibrosis replacing the normal areolar and vascular tissue (Arenberg, Marowitz and Shambaugh, 1970; Gussen, 1971b; Hallpike and Cairns, 1938). The vestibular aqueduct may be narrowed; it may fail to be visualized on radiographic study (Clemis and Valvassori, 1968; Pulec, 1972).

An experimental correlate for the distention of the cochlear duct in Meniere's syndrome is the production of endolymphatic hydrops through obliteration of the endolymphatic sac or obstruction of the vestibular aqueduct or endolymphatic duct (Beal, 1968;

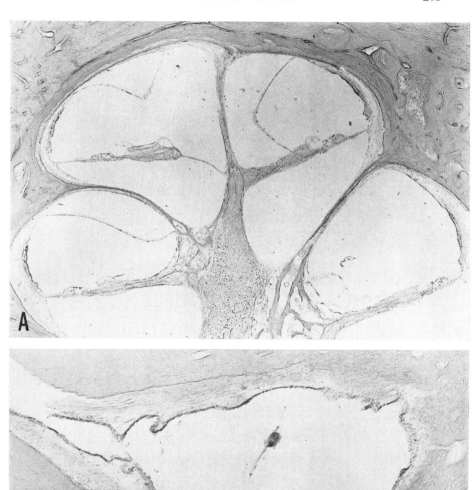

Figure 89. Meniere's syndrome.
Figure 89A. Endolympatic hydrops is severe.
Figure 89B. An unusual finding in the form of a dilated endolymphatic sac with obliteration of rugae. There is hyaline fibrosis of the subepithelial stroma.

Temporal bone courtesy Dr. Morgan Berthrong.

Kimura, 1967, 1968; Kimura, Schuknecht and Ota, 1974; Suh and Cody, 1974). There is variation in the foregoing effect among species, the guinea pig appearing most susceptible, and degree of hydrops increases with duration of experiment.

The question of degeneration of sensorineural elements in Meniere's syndrome has received considerable attention. Negative

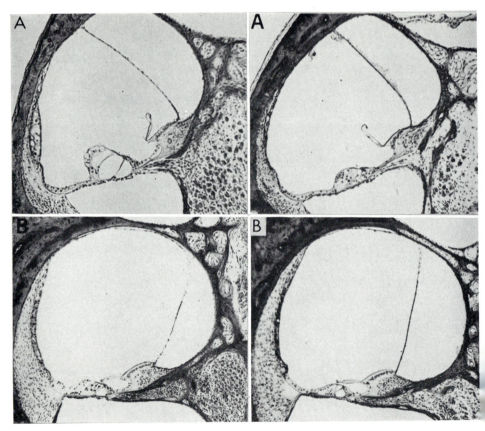

Figure 90. Experimental endolymphatic hydrops, guinea pig.
Left. Eleven months postop. A. Apical turn showing (in addition to the hydrops) edematous stria vascularis and loss of two rows of outer hair cells. B. Basal turn. Sensory cells and stria remain normal.
Right. Thirteen months postop. A. Apical turn showing atrophy of stria vascularis, sensory cells and spiral ganglion. B. Basal turn. Degeneration of outer sensory cells and spiral ganglion.
Illustrations courtesy Kimura, *Ann Otol,76*:664, 1967.

findings have been felt by some to require consideration of biochemical alterations as being of paramount pathophysiological import. It can be observed comparatively, however, that in glaucoma, temporary dysfunction attendant on increased hydrostatic pressure, with interim remission on decrease of pressure, may produce increments of tissue injury resulting ultimately in optic atrophy. The same appears to be true of Meniere's syndrome. Structurally evident injury of the elements of the cochlear duct cannot reasonably serve as correlate of fluctuating hearing loss; however, if the process continues, degeneration of hair cells, cochlear neurons and, variably, stria vascularis, may become apparent. These changes have been observed in humans in severe cases and in late stages, when hearing loss has become irreversible (Hallpike and Cairns, 1938; House, 1968; Kohut and Lindsay, 1972; Lindsay, 1968; McCabe and Ryu, 1968).

The degeneration of the sensorineural elements of the cochlear duct in the presence of endolymphatic hydrops has been confirmed experimentally especially in long-term circumstances, in cats, but particularly in guinea pigs (Kimura, 1968; Kimura, Schuknecht, and Ota, 1974; Kristensen, 1961; Suh and Cody, 1974).

Vertigo of central origin and based on vascular insufficiency may be observed (Hallpike, 1962). This exemplifies the need for whole-auditory-pathway studies; such pertinent pathologic observations are yet to be provided. Vestibular neuronitis is characteristically unassociated with deficiency of hearing (Hallpike, 1962).

REFERENCES

Adams, G.L., Paparella, M.M., and El Fiky, F.M.: Primary and metastatic tumors of the temporal bone. *Laryngoscope, 81:*1273, 1971.

Adams, R.D.: Occlusion of the anterior inferior cerebellar artery. *Arch Neurol Psychiatr., 49:*765, 1943.

Aidin, R., Corner, B. and Tovey, G.: Kernicterus and prematurity. *Lancet, 1:*1153, 1950.

Alford, B.R., Shaver, E.F., Rosenberg, J.J. *et al.:* Physiologic and histopathologic effects of micro-embolism of the internal auditory artery. *Trans Am Otol Soc, 53:*110, 1965.

Alport, A.C.: Hereditary familial congenital haemorrhagic nephritis. *Br Med J, 1:*504, 1927.

Altmann, F.: Histopathology and etiology of otosclerosis: a critical review. In Schuknecht, H.F. (Ed.) : *Otosclerosis.* Boston, Little, 1962.

Altmann, F.: Postmeningitic labyrinth ossification with stapes fixation. *Arch Otolaryngol, 82:*470, 1965.

Ames, M.D., Plotkin, S.A., Wincheater, R.A. *et al.:* Central auditory imperception. A significant factor in congenital rubella deafness. *J A M A, 213:*419, 1970.

Amjad, A.H., Scheer, A.A., and Rosenthal, J.: Human internal auditory canal. *Arch Otolaryngol, 89:*709, 1969.

Andrew, W.: Structural alterations with aging in the nervous system. *Proc Assoc Res Nerv Ment Dis, 35:*129, 1956.

Angelborg, C., and Engström, H.: Supporting elements in the organ of Corti. Fibrillar structures in the supporting cells of the organ of Corti of mammals. *Acta Otolaryngol, Suppl,* 301, 1972.

Anson, B.J., Warpeha, R.L., Donaldson, J.A., *et al.:* The developmental and adult anatomy of the membranous and osseous labyrinths of the otic capsule. *Otolaryngol Clin N Am,* Oct, 1968.

Arenberg, I.K., Marovitz, W.F., and Shambaugh, G.E., Jr.: The role of the endolymphatic sac in the pathogenesis of endolymphatic hydrops in man. *Acta Otolaryngol, Suppl, 275:*1970.

Arey, L.B.: *Developmental Anatomy,* Ed. VII. Philadelphia, Saunders, 1965.

Armed Forces Institute of Pathology: In Luna, L.G. (Ed.): *Manual of Histologic Staining Methods,* Ed. III. New York, McGraw, 1968.

Axelsson, A.: The vascular anatomy of the cochlea in the guinea pig and in man. *Acta Otolaryngol, Suppl, 243:*1968.

Axelsson, A., Miller, J., and Holmquist, J.: Studies of cochlear vasculature and sensory structures: A modified method. *Ann. Otol, 83:*537, 1974.

Balogh, K., Jr., Draskoczy, P.R., and Caulfield, J.B.: Norepinephrine in tumors of the jugular glomus. *Am J Pathol, 48:*1063, 1966.

Barnes, W.T., Magoun, H.W., and Ranson, S.W.: The ascending auditory pathway in the brain stem of the monkey. *J Comp Neurol, 79:*129, 1943.

Bast, T., and Anson, B.J.: *The Temporal Bone and The Ear.* Springfield, Thomas, 1949.

Beal, D.D.: Effect of endolymphatic sac ablation in the rabbit and cat. *Acta Otolaryngol, 66:*333, 1968.

Beal, D.D., Davey, P.R., and Lindsay, J.R.: Inner ear pathology of congenital deafness. *Arch Otolaryngol, 85:*134, 1967.

Beal, D.D., Hemenway, W.G., and Lindsay, J.R.: Inner ear pathology of sudden deafness. Histopathology of acquired deafness in the adult coincident with viral infection. *Arch Otolaryngol, 85:*591, 1967.

Belluci, R.J., Fisher, E.G., and Rhodin, J.: Ultrastructure of the round window membrane. *Laryngoscope 82:*1021, 1972.

Birge, E.A., and Imhoff, C.E.: Versenate as a decalcifying agent for bone. *Am J Clin Pathol, 22:*192, 1952.

Blanc, W.A., and Johnson, L.: Studies on kernicterus. Relationship with sulfonamide intoxication. Report on kernicterus in rats with glucuronyl transferase deficiency and review of pathogenesis. *J Neuropathol Exp Neurol, 18:*165, 1959.

Bloom, W., and Fawcett, D. W.: *A Textbook of Histology,* Ed. IX. Philadelphia, Saunders, 1968.

Bohne, B.A.: Location of small cochlear lesions by phase contrast microscopy prior to thin sectioning. *Laryngoscope, 82:*1, 1972.

Bredberg, G.: Cellular pattern and nerve supply of the human organ of Corti. *Acta Otolaryngol, Suppl, 236,* 1968.

Bredberg, G., Ades, H.W., and Engström, H.: Scanning electron microscopy of the normal and pathologically altered organ of Corti. *Acta Otolaryngol, Suppl, 301,* 1972.

Brody, H.: Organization of the cerebral cortex. Study of aging in human cerebral cortex. *J Comp Neurol, 102:*511, 1955.

Brummett, R.E., Himes, D., Saine, B. *et al.:* A comparative study of the ototoxicity of tobramycin and gentamycin. *Arch Otolaryngol, 96:*505, 1972.

Buch, N.H., Tygstrup, I., and Jörgensen, M.B.: Erythroblastosis fetalis and the hearing organ. *Acta Otolaryngol, 61:*387, 1966.

Byers, R.K., Paine, R.S., and Crothers, B.: Extrapyramidal cerebral palsy with hearing loss following erythroblastosis. *Ped, 15:*248, 1955.

Cammermeyer, J.: The postmortem origin and mechanism of neuronal hyperchromatosis and nuclear pyknosis. *Exp Neurol, 2:*379, 1960.

Carhart, R.: Cochlear otosclerosis: Audiological considerations. *Ann Otol, 75:*559, 1966.

Carhart, R.: Probable mechanisms underlying kernicteric hearing loss. *Acta Otolaryngol, Suppl 221,* 1967a.

Carhart, R.: Audiologic tests: Questions and speculations. In McConnell, F. and Ward, P.H. (Eds.): *Deafness in Childhood.* Nashville, Vanderbilt U Pr, 1967b.

Carruthers, D.G.: Congenital deaf-mutism as a sequela of a rubella-like maternal infection during pregnancy. *Med J Australia, 1:*315, 1945.

Cavanaugh, F.: The rhesus factor in deafness. *J Laryngol, 68:*444, 1954.

Chen, H., Wang, C., Tsan, K. *et al.:* An electron microscopic and radio-autographic study on experimental kernicterus. *Am J Pathol, 48:*683, 1966.

Chevance, L.G., Causse, J., Bretlau, P. *et al.:* Hydrolytic activity of the perilymph in otosclerosis. *Acta Otolaryngol, 74:*23, 1972.

Clemis, J.D.: Allergic cochleovestibular disturbances. *Trans Am Acad Ophthalmol Otolaryngol, 76:*1451, 1972.

Clemis, J.D., Boyles, J., Harford, E.R. *et al.:* The clinical diagnosis of Paget's disease of the temporal bone. *Ann Otol, 76:*611, 1967.

Clemis, J.D., and Valvassori, G.E.: Recent radiographic and clinical observations on the vestibular aqueduct. *Otolaryngol Clin N Am,* Oct, 1968.

Cohen, P.: Rh child: deaf or "aphasic?": "Aphasia" in kernicterus. *J Speech Hear Disord, 21:*411, 1956.

Cohn, A.M., Sataloff, J., and Lindsay, J.R.: Histiocytosis X (Letterer-Siwe disease) with involvement of the inner ear. *Arch Otolaryngol, 91:*24, 1970.

Comis, S.D., and Whitfield, I.C.: Centrifugal excitation and inhibition in the cochlear nucleus. *J Physiol, 188:*34, 1967.

Crabtree, N., and Gerrard, J.: Perceptive deafness associated with severe neonatal jaundice. *J Laryngol Otol, 64:*482, 1950.

Crigler, J.F., Jr., and Najjar, V.A.: Congenital familial nonhemolytic jaundice with kernicterus. *Ped, 10:*169, 1952.

Crysdale, W.S., and Stahle, J.: Ultrasonic irradiation of the guinea pig cochlea. *Ann Otol, 81:*87, 1972.

Davis, G.L.: Cytomegalovirus in the inner ear. *Ann Otol, 78:*1179, 1969.

Day, R.L.: Experimental and clinical observations of hyperbilirubinemia. In *Kernicterus and its Importance in Cerebral Palsy.* Springfield, Thomas, 1961.

Dayal, V.S.: A study of crossed olivocochlear bundle on adaptation of auditory action potentials. *Laryngoscope 82:*693, 1972.

de Lorenzo, A.J.: The fine structure of synapses in the ciliary ganglion of the chick. *J Biophys Biochem Cytol, 7:*31, 1960a.

de Lorenzo, A.J.D.: Electron microscopic observations of the auditory cortex with particular reference to synaptic junctions. In Rasmussen, G.L., and Windle, W.F.: (Eds.): *Neural Mechanisms of the Auditory and Vestibular Systems.* Springfield, Thomas, 1960b.

de Lorenzo, A.J.D., Shirokyd, V., and Cohn, E.I.: Distribution of exogenous horseradish peroxidase in perilymphatic and endolymphatic spaces of the guinea pig cochlea. In de Lorenzo, A.J.D. (Ed.) : *Vascular Disorders and Hearing Defects.* Baltimore, Univ Park Pr, 1973.

Densert, O., and Flock, A.: An electron-microscopic study of adrenergic innervation in the cochlea. *Acta Otolaryngol, 77*:185, 1974.

Dix, M.R.: Observations upon the nerve fiber deafness of multiple sclerosis with particular reference to the phenomenon of loudness recruitment. *J Laryngol, 79*:695, 1965.

Dix, M.R., and Hood, J.D.: Symmetrical hearing loss in brain stem lesions. Acta Otolaryngol, 75:165, 1973.

Donahue, D., and Gussen, R.: Rapid parlodion embedding of temporal bones. *Arch Otolaryngol, 83*:54, 1966.

Donaldson, J.A., and Miller, J.M.: Anatomy of the inner ear. In Paparella, M.M., and Shumrick, D.A. (Eds.) : *Otolaryngology.* Philadelphia, Saunders, 1973.

Dublin, W.B.: Metastasizing intracranial tumors. *Northwest Med, 43*:83, 1944a.

Dublin, W.B.: Combined Bodian and Masson staining method applied to skin. *Arch Derm Syph, 50*:361, 1944b.

Dublin, W.B.: Pathogenesis of kernicterus. *J Neuropathol Exp Neurol, 8*: 119, 1949.

Dublin, W.B.: Neurologic lesions of erythroblastosis fetalis in relation to nuclear deafness. *Am J Clin Pathol, 21*:935, 1951.

Dublin, W.B.: *Fundamentals of Neuropathology,* Ed. II Springfield, Thomas, 1967.

Dublin, W.B.: Cytoarchitecture of the cochlear nuclei. Report of an illustrative case of erythroblastosis. *Arch Otolaryngol, 100*:355, 1974.

Duke, W.W., Boshell, B.R., Soteres, P. *et al.*: A norepinephrine-secreting glomus jugulare tumor presenting as a pheochromocytoma. *Ann Int Med, 60*:1040, 1964.

Duvall, A.J., III, and Sutherland, C.R.: Cochlear transport of horseradish peroxidase. *Ann Otol, 81*:705, 1972.

Edmonds, C., Freeman, P., and Tonkin, J.: Fistula of the round window in diving. *Trans Am Acad Opthalmol Otolaryngol, 78*:444, 1974.

Engström, H., Ades, H.W., and Andersson, A.: *Structural Pattern of the Organ of Corti.* Baltimore, Williams & Wilkins, 1966.

Engström, H., Ades, H.W., and Bredberg, G.: Normal structure of the organ of Corti and the effect of noise-induced cochlear damage. In Wolstenholme, G.E.W., Knight, J. (Eds.): *Sensorineural Hearing Loss.* London, J. and A. Churchill, 1970.

Engström, H., and Kohonen, A.: Cochlear damage from ototoxic antibiotics. *Acta Otolaryngol, 59*:171, 1965.

Engström, H., and Röckert, H.: Normal histology of the labyrinthine capsule and oval window area. In Schuknecht, H.F. (Ed.): *Otosclerosis.* Boston, Little, 1962.

Engström, H., and Wersäll, J.: Is there a special nutritive cellular system around the hair cells in the organ of Corti? *Ann Otol, 62*:507, 1953.

Ernster, L., Herlin, L., and Zetterström, R.: Experimental studies on the pathogenesis of kernicterus. *Ped, 20*:647, 1957.

Fairbanks, D.N.F., Wallenberg, E.A., and Webb, B.M.: Acupuncture for hearing loss. *Arch Otolaryngol, 99*:395, 1974.

Falbe-Hansen, J., Christensen, E., Gisselsson, L. *et al.*: Effect of acute and prolonged oxygen deprivation on the organ of Corti in guinea pigs and cats. *Arch Otolaryngol, 67*:71, 1958.

Fernandez, C.: Postmortem changes and artifacts in human temporal bones. *Laryngoscope, 68*:1586, 1958.

Fernandez, C., and Karapas, F.: The course and termination of the striae of Monakow and Held in the cat. *J Comp Neurol, 131*:371, 1967.

Fisch, L.: The aetiology of congenital deafness and audiometric patterns. *J Laryngol, 69*:479, 1955.

Fisch, U., Dobozi, M., and Greig, D.: Degenerative changes of the arterial vessels of the internal auditory meatus during the process of aging. *Acta Otolaryngol, 73*:259, 1972.

Flottorp, G., Morley, D.E., and Skatvedt, M.: The localization of hearing impairment in athetoids. *Acta Otolaryngol, 48*:404, 1957.

Forster, F.M., and McCormack, R.A.: Kernicterus unassociated with erythroblastosis fetalis. *J Neuropathol Exp Neurol, 3*:379, 1944.

Fujita, S., and Hayden, R.C., Jr.: Alport's syndrome. Temporal bone report. *Arch Otolaryngol, 90*:453, 1969.

Gacek, R.R., Nomura, Y., and Balogh, K.: Acetylcholinesterase activity in the efferent fibers of the stato-acoustic nerve. *Acta Otolaryngol, 59*:541, 1965.

Gacek, R.R., and Schuknecht, H.F.: Pathology of presbycusis. *Intl Audiol, 8*:199, 1969.

Gaeth, J.: Study of phonemic regression in relation to hearing loss. Thesis, Northwestern University, Chicago, 1948, quoted by Schuknecht, 1974.

Galambos, R.: Suppression of auditory nerve activity by stimulation of efferent fibers to cochlea. *J Neurophysiol, 19*:424, 1956.

Gamble, J.E., Peterson, E.A., and Chandler, J.R.: Radiation effects on the inner ear. *Arch Otolaryngol, 88*:156, 1968.

Geniec, P., and Morest, D.K.: The neuronal architecture of the human posterior colliculus. *Acta Otolaryngol, Suppl, 295*, 1971.

Gerrard, J.: Nuclear jaundice and deafness. *J Laryngol, 66*:39, 1952.

Gillilan, L.A.: The correlation of the blood supply to the human brain stem with clinical brain stem lesions. *J Neuropathol Exp Neurol, 23*:78, 1964.

Goldberg, J.M., and Brown, P.B.: Functional organization of the dog superior olivary complex: An anatomical and electrophysiological study. *J Neurophysiol, 31*:639, 1968.

Goldberg, J.M., and Moore, R.Y.: Ascending projections of the lateral lemniscus in the cat and monkey. *J Comp Neurol, 129*:143, 1967.

Gonzalez, G., Miller, N., and Wasilewski, V.: Progressive neuro-ototoxicity of kanamycin. *Ann Otol, 81*:127, 1972.

Gonzalez-Revilla, A.: Neurinomas of the cerebellopontine recess; clinical study of 160 cases including operative mortality and end results. *Bull Johns Hopkins Hosp, 80*:254, 1947.

Gonzalez-Revilla, A.: Differential diagnosis of tumors at the cerebellopontile recess. *Bull Johns Hopkins Hosp, 83*:187, 1948.

Gooch, J.M.: Neurologic sequelae of jaundice of prematurity. *Med J Australia, 48*:117, 1961.

Gray, H.: In Goss, C.M. (Ed.): *Anatomy of the Human Body,* Ed. XXVIII. Philadelphia, Lea & Febiger, 1966.

Guild, S.R.: A graphic reconstruction method for the study of the organ of Corti. *Anat Rec, 22*:141, 1921.

Guild, S.R.: Observations upon the structure and normal contents of the ductus and saccus endolymphaticus in the guinea-pig (*Cavia cobaya*). The circulation of the endolymph. *Am J Anat, 39*:1, 57, 1927.

Guild, S.R.: Correlations of histologic observations and the acuity of hearing. *Acta Otolaryngol, 17*:207, 1932.

Guild, S.R.: Comments oin the physiology of hearing and the anatomy of the inner ear. *Laryngoscope, 47*:365, 1937.

Guild, S.R.: A hitherto unrecognized structure, the glomus jugulare, in man. *Anat Rec, 79*:Suppl. 2, 1941.

Gussen, R.: Intramodiolar acoustic neurinoma. *Laryngoscope, 81*:1979, 1971a.

Gussen, R.: Tissue changes about the endolymphatic sac. *Arch Ototolaryngol, 94*:406, 1971b.

Gussen, R.: Malnutrition and deafness. *J Laryngol, 88*:523, 1974.

Hall, J.G.: The cochlea and the cochlear nuclei in neonatal asphyxia. *Acta Otolaryngol, Suppl, 194,* 1964.

Hall, J.G.: The cochlea and cochlear nuclei in the bat (Plecotus auritus), *Acta Otolaryngol, 67*:490, 1969.

Hallpike, C.S.: Vertigo of central origin. *Proc Roy Soc Med, 55*:364, 1962.

Hallpike, C.S.: The loudness recruitment phenomenon: A clinical contribution to the neurology of hearing. In Graham, A.B. (Ed.): *Sensorineural Hearing Processes and Disorders.* Boston, Little, 1967.

Hallpike, C.S., and Cairns, H.: Observations on the pathology of Meniere's syndrome. *J Laryngol, 53*:625, 1938.

Hansen, C.C.: Perceptive hearing loss and increased intracranial pressure. *Arch Otolaryngol, 87*:63, 1968a.

Hansen, C.C.: Perceptive hearing loss and arterial hypertension. *Arch Otolaryngol, 87*:119, 1968b.

Hawkins, J.E., Jr.: The role of vasoconstriction in noise-induced hearing loss. *Ann Otol, 80*:903, 1971.

Hawkins, J.E., Jr., Johnsson, L.G., and Preston, R.F.: Cochlear microvasculature in normal and damaged ears. *Laryngoscope, 82:*1091, 1972.

Hilding, D.A.: Cochlear chromaffin cells. *Laryngoscope, 75:*1, 1965.

Hinojosa, R.: Transport of ferritin across Reissner's membrane. *Acta Otolaryngol, Suppl, 292,* 1971.

Hinojosa, R., and Rodriguez-Echandia, E.L.: The fine structure of the stria vascularis of the cat inner ear. *Am J Anat, 118:*631, 1966.

Hitselberger, W.E., and Gardner, G., Jr.: Other tumors of the cerebellopontine angle. *Arch Otolaryngol, 88:*712, 1968.

Holden, H.B., and Schuknecht, H.F.: Distribution pattern of blood in the inner ear following spontaneous subarachnoid hemorrhage. *J Laryngal, 82:*321, 1968.

Honrubia, V., Strelioff, D., and Ward, P.H.: The mechanism of excitation of the hair cells in the cochlea. *Laryngoscope, 81:*1719, 1971.

Hough, J.V.D.: Otologic trauma. In Paparella, M.M., and Shumrick, D.A. (Eds.): *Otolaryngology.* Philadelphia, Saunders, 1973.

House, W.F.: A theory of the production of symptoms of Meniere's disease. *Otolaryngol Clin N Am,* Oct, 1968.

Igarashi, M.: Pathology of the inner ear end organs. In Minckler, J. (Ed.): *Pathology of the Nervous System.* New York, McGraw, 1972.

Igarashi, M., Alford, B.R., Nakai, Y. *et al.:* Behavioral auditory function after transection of crossed olivo-cochlear bundle in the cat. *Acta Otolaryngol, 73:*455, 1972.

Igarashi, M., Saito, R., Alford, B.R. *et al.:* Temporal bone findings in pneumoccocal meningitis. *Arch Otolaryngol, 99:*79, 1974.

Illum, P.: The Mondini type of cochlear malformation. A survey of the literature. *Arch Otolaryngol, 96:*305, 1972.

Illum, P., Kiaer, H.W., Hvidberg-Hansen, J. *et al.:* Fifteen cases of Pendred's syndrome. Congenital deafness and sporadic goiter. *Arch Otolaryngol, 96:*297, 1972.

Irving, R., and Harrison, J.M.: The superior olivary complex and audition. *J Comp Neurol, 130:*77, 1967.

Iurato, S., Luciano, L., Pannese, E. *et al.:* Histochemical localization of acetylcholinesterase (AChE) activity in the inner ear. *Acta Otolaryngol, Suppl, 279,* 1971.

Jerger, J., Weikers, N.S., Sharbrough, F.W.. III *et al.:* Bilateral lesions of the temporal lobe. A case study. *Acta Otolaryngol, Suppl, 258,* 1969.

Johnson, E.W.: Audiologic diagnosis of acoustic neuromas. *Arch Otolaryngol, 89:*280, 1969.

Johnson, L., Garcia, M.L., Figueroa, E. *et al.:* Kernicterus in rats lacking glucuronyl transferase. *Am J Dis Child, 101:*322, 1961.

Johnsson, L.-G.: Reissner's membrane in the human cochlea. *Ann Otol, 80:* 425, 1971.

Johnsson, L.-G.: Sequence of degeneration of Corti's organ and its first-order neurons. *Ann Otol, 83:*294, 1974.

Johnsson, L.-G., and Hawkins, J.E., Jr.: A direct approach to cochlear anatomy and pathology in man. *Arch Otolaryngol, 85:*599, 1967.

Johnsson, L.-G., and Hawkins, J.E., Jr.: Strial atrophy in clinical and experimental deafness. *Laryngoscope, 82:*1105, 1972a.

Johnsson, L.-G., and Hawkins, J.E., Jr.: Sensory and neural degeneration with aging as seen in microdissections of the human inner ear. *Ann Otol, 81:*179, 1972b.

Johnsson, L.-G., and Hawkins, J.E., Jr.: Vascular changes in the human inner ear associated with aging. *Ann Otol, 81:*364, 1972c.

Jordan, V.M., Pinheiro, M.L., Chiba, K. *et al.:* Postmortem changes in surface preparations of the cochlea. *Ann Otol, 82:*111, 1973.

Jörgensen, M.B.: Changes of aging in the inner ear, and the inner ear in diabetes mellitus. Histological studies. *Acta Otolaryngol Suppl, 188,* 1964.

Jörgensen, M.B., and Kristensen, H.K.: Irradiation and otosclerosis. Histological studies. *Ann Otol, 75:*677, 1966.

Kaku, Y., Farmer, J.C., Jr., and Hudson, W.R.: Ototoxic drug effects on cochlear histochemistry. *Arch Otolaryngol, 98:*282, 1973.

Kao, F.F., Baker, R.H., Jr., Leung, S.J. *et al.:* Efficacy of acupuncture for the treatment of sensorineural deafness. *Am J Chinese Med, 1:*283, 1973.

Karlan, M.S., Basek, M., and Potter, G.B.: Intracochlear neurilemoma. *Arch Otolaryngol, 96:*573, 1972.

Karmody, C.S.: Asymptomatic maternal rubella and congenital deafness. *Arch Otolaryngol, 89:*720, 1969.

Karmody, C.S., and Schuknecht, H.F.: Deafness in congenital syphilis. *Arch Otolaryngol, 83:*18, 1966.

Kelemen, G.: Toxoplasmosis and congenital deafness. *Arch Otolaryngol, 68:* 547, 1958.

Kelemen, G., Laor, Y., and Klein, E.: Laser induced ear damage. *Arch Otolaryngol, 86:*603, 1967.

Kelemen, G., and Linthicum, F.H., Jr.: Labyrinthine otosclerosis. *Acta Otolaryngol, Suppl, 253,* 1969.

Kellerhals, B., Engström, H., and Ades, H.W.: Die Morphologie des Ganglion spirale cochleae. (Abstract in English) *Acta Otolaryngol, Suppl, 226,* 1967.

Kiang, N.Y.: Stimulus coding in the auditory nerve and cochlear nucleus. *Acta Otolaryngol, 59:*186, 1965.

Kiang, N.Y., Pfeiffer, R.R., Warr, W.B., *et al.:* Stimulus coding in the cochlear nucleus. *Ann Otol, 74:*463, 1965.

Kiang, N.Y., Watanabe, T., Thomas, E.C., *et al.:* Stimulus coding in the cat's auditory nerve. *Ann Otol, 71:*1009, 1962.

Kimura, R.S.: Hairs of the cochlear sensory cells and their attachment to the tectorial membrane. *Acta Otolaryngol, 61:*55, 1966.

Kimura, R.S.: Experimental blockage of the endolymphatic duct and sac and its effect on the inner ear of the guinea pig. *Ann Otol, 76:*664, 1967.

Kimura, R.S.: Experimental production of endolymphatic hydrops. *Oto-*

laryngol Clin N Am, Oct. 1968.

Kimura, R.S., and Ota, C.Y.: Ultrastructure of the cochlear blood vessels. *Acta Otolaryngol, 77:*231, 1974.

Kimura, R.S., and Perlman, H.B.: Extensive venous obstruction of the labyrinth. Cochlear changes. *Ann Otol, 65:*332, 1956.

Kimura, R.S., and Perlman, H.B.: Arterial obstruction of the labyrinth. Cochlear changes. *Ann Otol, 67:*5, 1958.

Kimura, R.S., Schuknecht, H.F., and Ota, C.Y.: Blockage of the cochlear aqueduct. *Acta Otolaryngol, 77:*1, 1974.

Kimura, R.S., Schuknecht, H.F., and Sando, I.: Fine morphology of the sensory cells in the organ of Corti of man. *Acta Otolaryngol, 58:*390, 1964.

Kimura, R.S., and Wersäll, J.: Termination of the olivocochlear bundle in relation to the outer hair cells of the organ of Corti in guinea pig. *Acta Otolaryngol, 55:*11, 1962.

Kirikae, I., Sato, T., and Shitara, T.: Study of hearing in advanced age. *Laryngoscope, 74:*205, 1964.

Kohonen, A.: Effect of some ototoxic drugs upon the pattern and innervation of cochlear sensory cells in the guinea pig. *Acta Otolaryngol, Suppl, 208,* 1965.

Kohut, R.I., and Lindsay, J.R.: Pathologic changes in idiopathic labyrinthine hydrops. *Acta Otolaryngol, 73:*402, 1972.

Konigsmark, B.W.: Hereditary deafness in man. *N Engl J Med, 281:*713, 774, 827, 1969.

Konigsmark, B.W.: Hereditary deafness with external ear abnormalities. A review. *Johns Hopkins Med J, 127:*228, 1970.

Konigsmark, B.W.: Cellular organization of the cochlear nuclei in man. (Abstract) *J Neuropathol Exp Neurol, 32:*153, 1973.

Konigsmark, B.W., and Murphy, E.A.: Volume of the ventral cochlear nucleus in man: Its relationship to neuronal population and age. *J Neuropathol Exp Neurol, 31:*304, 1972.

Kos, A.O., Schuknecht, H.F., and Singer, J.D.: Temporal bone studies in 13 15 and 18 trisomy syndromes. *Arch Otolaryngol, 83:*439, 1966.

Kristensen, H.K.: Histopathology in Meniere's disease. *Acta Otolaryngol, 53:*237, 1961.

Krmpotic-Nemanic, J., Nemanic, D., and Kostovic, I.: Macroscopical and microscopical changes in the bottom of the internal auditory meatus. *Acta Otolaryngol, 73:*254, 1972.

Kuhn, F.A., Thalmann, R., and Marovitz, W.F.: A comparison of Nomarski differential interference contrast and phase contrast microscopy of the guinea pig organ of Corti. *Laryngoscope, 81:*1090, 1971.

La Ferriere, K.A., Arenberg, I.K., Hawkins, J.E., Jr. *et al.:* Melanocytes of the vestibular labyrinth and their relationship to the microvasculature. *Ann Otol, 83:*685, 1974.

Larsson, A.: Genetic problems in otosclerosis. In Schuknecht, H.F. (Ed.): *Otosclerosis.* Boston, Little, 1962.

Lawrence, M.: Some physiological factors in inner ear deafness. *Ann Otol,* 69:480, 1960.

Lawrence, M.: Histological evidence for localized radial flow of endolymph. *Arch Otolaryngol, 83:*406, 1966a.

Lawrence, M.: Possible influence of cochlear otosclerosis on inner ear fluids. *Ann Otol, 75:*553, 1966b.

Lawrence, M.: Effects of interference with terminal blood supply on organ of Corti. *Laryngoscope, 76:*1318, 1966c.

Lawrence, M.: Dynamics of labyrinthine fluids. *Arch Otolaryngol, 89:*85, 1969.

Lawrence, M.: Direct visualization of living organ of Corti and studies of its extracellular fluids. *Laryngoscope, 84:*1767, 1974.

Lawrence, M., and McCabe, B.F.: Inner ear mechanics and deafness. Special consideration of Menieres syndrome. *J A M A, 171:*1927, 1959.

Lawrence, M., and Wever, E.G.: Effects of oxygen deprivation upon the structure of the organ of Corti. *Arch Otolargnol, 55:*31, 1952.

Lebo, C.P., and Redell, R.C.: The presbycusis component in occupational hearing loss. *Laryngoscope, 82:*1399, 1972.

von Leden, H., and Horton, B.T.: Auditory nerve in multiple sclerosis. *Arch Otolaryngol, 48:*51, 1948.

Lenn, N.J., and Reese, T.S.: The fine structure of nerve endings in the nucleus of the trapezoid body and the ventral cochlear nucleus. *Am J Anat, 118:*375, 1966.

Leonard, J.R., and Talbot, M.L.: Asymptomatic acoustic neurilemoma. *Arch Otolaryngol, 91:*117, 1970.

Le Zak, R.J., and Selhub, S.: On hearing in multiple sclerosis. *Ann Otol, 75:*1102, 1966.

Liden, G.: The scope and application of current audiometric tests. *J Laryngol, 83:*507, 1969.

Lim, D.L.: Fine morphology of the tectorial membrane. *Arch Otolaryngol, 96:*199, 1972.

Lim, D.J., and Lane, W.C.: Three-dimensional observation of the inner ear with the scanning electron microscope. *Trans Am Acad Ophthalmol Otolaryngol, 73:*842, 1969.

Lim, D.J., and Melnick, W.: Acoustic damage of the cochlea. A scanning and transmission electron microscopic observation. *Arch Otolaryngol, 94:* 294, 1971.

Lindsay, J.R.: Sudden deafness due to virus infection. *Arch Otolaryngol, 69:*13, 1959.

Lindsay, J.R.: Histopathology of Meniere's disease as observed by light microscopy. *Otolaryngol Clin N Am,* Oct, 1968.

Lindsay, J.R.: Profound childhood deafness. Inner ear pathology. *Ann Otol, 82:* Suppl. 5, 1973a.

Lindsay, J.R.: Histopathology of otosclerosis. *Arch Otolaryngol, 97:*24, 1973b.

Lindsay, J.R.: *Otosclerosis.* In Paparella, M.M., and Schumrick, D.A. (Eds.):

Otolaryngology. Philadelphia, Saunders, 1973c.

Lindsay, J.R., Carruthers, D.G., Hemenway, W.G. *et al.:* Inner ear pathology following maternal rubella. *Ann Otol, 62:*1201, 1953.

Lindsay, J.R., Davey, P.R., and Ward, P.H.: Inner ear pathology in deafness due to mumps. *Ann Otol, 69:*918, 1960.

Lindsay, J.R., and Hemenway, W.G.: Inner ear pathology due to measles. *Ann Otol, 63:*754, 1954.

Linthicum, F.H., Jr.: Correlation of sensorineural hearing impairment and otosclerosis. *Ann Otol, 75:*512, 1966.

Linthicum, F.H., Jr.: Diagnosis of cochlear otosclerosis. *Arch Otolaryngol, 95:*564, 1972.

Lipscomb, D.M., and Roettger, R.L.: Capillary constriction in cochlear and vestibular tissues during intense noise stimulation. *Laryngoscope, 83:*259, 1973.

Logan, T.B., Prazma, J., Thomas, W.G. *et al.:* Tobramycin ototoxicity. *Arch Otolaryngol, 99:*190, 1974.

Lopez-Rios, G., Benitez, J.T., and Vivar, G.: Histiocytosis: Histopathological study of the temporal bone. *Ann Otol, 77:*1171, 1969.

Lorente de No, R.: Anatomy of the eighth nerve. The central projection of the nerve endings of the internal ear. *Laryngoscope, 43:*1, 1933a.

Lorente de No, R.: Anatomy of the eighth nerve. General plan of structure of the primary cochlear nuclei. *Laryngoscope, 43:*327, 1933b.

Lorente de No, R.: The sensory endings in the cochlea. *Laryngoscope, 47:*373, 1937.

Lundquist, P.-G.: The endolymphatic duct and sac in the guinea pig. An electron microscopic and experimental investigation. *Acta Otolaryngol, Suppl, 201,* 1965.

Maniglia, A.J., Wolff, D., and Herques, A.J.: Congenital deafness in 13-15 trisomy syndrome. *Arch Otolaryngol, 92:*181, 1970.

Marcus, R.E., and Goldenberg, R.A.: Cochleoneural hearing loss treated with acupuncture. *Arch Otolaryngol, 99:*451, 1974.

Massopust, L.C., Jr., and Ordy, J.M.: Auditory organization of the inferior colliculi in the cat. *Exp Neurol, 6:*465, 1962.

Matkin, N.D., and Carhart, R.: Auditory profiles associated with Rh incompatibility. *Arch Otolaryngol, 84:*502, 1966.

Matschinsky, F.M., and Thalmann, R.: Energy metabolism of the cochlear duct. In Paparella, M.M. (Ed.): *Biochemical Mechanisms in Hearing and Deafness.* Springfield, Thomas 1970.

Mawson, S.R.: *Diseases of the Ear.* Boston, Williams and Wilkins, 1963.

McCabe, B.F., and Ryu, J.H.: Pathophysiology of the vertiginous episode in Meniere's disease. *Otolaryngol Clin N Am,* Oct, 1968.

McCabe, B.F., and Wolsk, D.: Experimental inner ear pressure changes. *Ann Otol, 70:*541, 1961.

McDonald, D.M., and Rasmussen, G.L.: Association of acetylcholinesterase with one type of synaptic ending in the cochlear nucleus: An electron microscopic study. (Abstract) *Anat Rec, 163*:228, 1969.

McDonald, D.M., and Rasmussen, G.L.: Ultrastructural characteristics of synaptic endings in the cochlear nucleus having acetylcholinesterase activity. *Brain Res, 28*:1, 1971.

McGee, T.M., and Olszewski, J.: Streptomycin sulfate and dihydrostreptomycin ototoxicity. *Arch Otolaryngol, 75*:295, 1962.

McLay, K., and Maran, A.G.D.: Deafness and the Klippel-Feil syndrome. *J Laryngol, 83*:175, 1969.

Mendelsohn, M., and Katzenberg, I.: The effect of kanamycin on the cation content of the endolymph. *Laryngoscope, 82*:397, 1972.

Mendelsohn, M., and Roderique, J.: Cationic changes in endolymph during hypoglycemia. *Laryngoscope, 82*:1533, 1972.

Mendoza, D., Rius, M., De Stefani, E., and Leborgne, F., Jr.: Experimental otosclerosis. Its causation by ionizing radiations. *Acta Otolaryngol, 67*:9, 1969.

Meriwether, L.S., Hager, H., and Scholz, W.: Kernicterus. Hypoxemia, significant pathogenic factor. *Arch Neurol Psychiatry, 73*:293, 1955.

Meuwissen, H.J., and Robinson, G.C.: The ototoxic antibiotics. A survey of current knowledge. *Clin Ped, 6*:262, 1967.

Miller, G.W., Joseph, D.J., Cozad, R.L. *et al.:* Alport's syndrome. *Arch Otolaryngol, 92*:419, 1970.

Miller, M.H., Rabinowitz, M., and Cohen, M.: Pure-tone audiometry in prenatal rubella. *Arch Otolaryngol, 94*:25, 1971.

Minckler, J.: Communication disorders. In Minckler, J. (Ed.): *Pathology of the Nervous System.* New York, McGraw, 1972.

Mnich, Z.: Permeability of Reissner's membrane in this isolated ear of the guinea-pig. *Acta Otolaryngol, 71*:27, 1971.

Morest, D.K.: The neuronal architecture of the medial geniculate body of the cat. *J Anat, 98*:611, 1964.

Morest, D.K.: The laminar structure of the medial geniculate body of the cat. *J Anat, 99*:1, 1965.

Morest, D.K.: Dendrodendritic synapses of cells that have axons: The fine structure of the Golgi type II cell in the medial geniculate body of the cat. (In English) *Z Anat Entwickl-Gesch, 133*:216, 1971.

Morgenstein, K.M., and Manace, E.D.: Temporal bone histopathology in sickle cell disease. *Laryngoscope, 79*:2172, 1969.

Mountjoy, J.R., Dolan, K.D., and McCabe, B.F.: Neurilemmoma of the ninth cranial nerve masquerading as an acoustic neuroma. *Arch Otolaryngol, 100*:65, 1974.

Moushegian, G., Rupert, A., and Galambos, R.: Microelectrode study of ventral cochlear nucleus of the cat. *J Neurophysiology, 25*:515, 1962.

Myers, E.N., and Stool, S.: Cytomegalic inclusion disease of the inner ear. *Laryngoscope, 78*:1904, 1968.

Myers, G.J., and Tyler, H.R.: The etiology of deafness in Alport's syndrome. *Arch Otolaryngol, 96*:333, 1972.

Nager, G.T.: *Meningiomas Involving the Temporal Bone.* Springfield, Thomas, 1964a.

Nager, G.T.: Association of bilateral VIIIth nerve tumors with meningiomas in von Recklinghausen's disease. *Laryngoscope, 74:*1220, 1964b.

Nager, G.T.: Gliomas involving the temporal bone. Clinical and pathological aspects. *Laryngoscope, 77:*454, 1967.

Nager, G.T.: Acoustic neurinomas. Pathology and differential diagnosis. *Arch Otolaryngol, 89:*252, 1969a.

Nager, G.T.: Histopathology of otosclerosis. *Arch Otolaryngol, 89:*341, 1969b.

Nakai, Y., and Hilding, D.A.: Electron microscopic studies of adenosine triphosphatase activity in the stria vascularis and spiral ligament. *Acta Otolaryngol, 62:*411, 1966.

Neff, W.D.: Role of the auditory cortex in sound discrimination. In Rasmussen, G.L., and Windle, W.F. (Eds.): *Neural Mechanisms of the Auditory and Vestibular Systems.* Springfield, Thomas, 1960.

Noffsinger, D., Olsen, W.O., Carhart, R. *et al.:* Auditory and vestibular aberrations in multiple sclerosis. *Acta Otolaryngol, Suppl, 303, 1972.*

Ogura, Y., and Clemis, J.D.: A study of the gross anatomy of the human vestibular aqueduct. *Ann Otol, 80:*813, 1971.

Olszewski, J., and Baxter, D.: *Cytoarchitecture of the Human Brain Stem.* Philadelphia, Lippincott, 1954.

Osen, K.K.: The intrinsic organization of the cochlear nuclei in the cat. *Acta Otolaryngol, 67:*352, 1969a.

Osen, K.K.: Cytoarchitecture of the cochlear nuclei in the cat. *J Comp Neurol, 136:*453, 1969b.

Osen, K.K.: Course and termination of the primary afferents in the cochlear nuclei of the cat. (In English) *Arch Ital Biol, 108:*21, 1970.

Osen, K.K.: Projection of the cochlear nuclei on the inferior colliculus in the cat. *J Comp Neurol, 144:*355, 1972.

Osen, K.K., and Jansen, J.: The cochlear nuclei in the common porpoise, *Phocaena phocaena. J Comp Neurol, 125:*223, 1965.

Osen, K.K., and Roth, K.: Histochemical localization of cholinesterases in the cochlear nuclei of the cat, with notes on the origin of acetylcholinesterase-postive afferents and the superior olive. *Brain Res, 16:*165, 1969.

Palant, D.I., and Carter, B.L.: Klippel-Feil syndrome and deafness. *Am J Dis Child, 128:*218, 1972.

Pang, L.Q.: Sudden sensorineural hearing loss following diving and treatment by recompression: A report of two cases. *Trans Am Acad Ophthalmol Otolaryngol, 78:*436, 1974.

Paparella, M.M., and Capps, M.J.: Sensorineural deafness in children — Nongenetic. In Paparella, M.M., and Shumrick, D.A. (Eds.): *Otolaryngology.* Philadelphia, Saunders, 1973.

Paparella, M.M., and El Fiky, F.M.: Ear involvement in malignant lymphoma. *Ann Otol, 81:*352, 1972.

Paparella, M.M., Oda, M., Hiraide, F. *et al.:* Pathology of sensorineural hearing loss in otitis media. *Ann Otol, 81:*632, 1972.

Paparella, M.M., and Sugiura, S.: The pathology of suppurative labyrinthitis. *Ann Otol, 76:*554, 1967.

Peng, A.: Acupuncture treatment for deafness. *Am J. Chinese Med, 1:*155, 1974.

Perez de Moura, L.F., and Hayden, R.C., Jr.: Salicylate ototoxicity. A human temporal bone report. *Arch Otolaryngol, 87:*368, 1968.

Perlman, H.B.: Labyrinth capsule lesions with generalized disease of the skeleton. In Paparella, M.M., and Shumrick, D.A. (Eds.): *Otolaryngology.* Philadelphia, Saunders, 1973.

Perlman, H.B., and Kimura, R.S.: Observations of the living blood vessels of the cochlea. *Ann Otol, 64:*1176, 1955.

Perlman, H.B., and Kimura, R.S.: Experimental obstruction of venous drainage and arterial supply of the inner ear. *Ann Otol, 66:*537, 1957.

Polus, K.: The problem of vascular deafness. *Laryngoscope, 82:*24, 1972.

Powell, T.P.S., and Erulkar, S.D.: Transneuronal cell degeneration in the auditory relay nuclei of the cat. *J Anat, 96:*249, 1962.

Powers, W.H.: Metabolic aspects of Meniere's disease. *Laryngoscope, 82:*1716, 1972.

Powers, W.H.: Allergic factors in Meniere's disease. *Trans Am Acad Ophthalmol Otolaryngol, 77:*ORL22, 1973.

Priede, V.M., and Coles, R.R.A.: Interpretation of loudness recruitment tests — Some new concepts and criteria. *J Laryngol, 88:*641, 1974.

Proctor, B., Gurdjian, E.S., and Webster, J.E.: The ear in head trauma. *Laryngoscope, 66:*16, 1956.

Pujol, R., and Hilding, D.: Anatomy and physiology of the onset of auditory function. *Acta Otolaryngol, 76:*1, 1973.

Pulec, J.L. (Ed.): *Meniere's Disease.* Philadelphia, Saunders, 1968.

Pulec, J.L.: Meniere's disease. Results of a two and one-half-year study of etiology, natural history, and results of treatment. *Laryngoscope, 82:*1703, 1972.

Pullen, F.W., II: Round window membrane rupture: A cause of sudden deafness. *Trans Am Acad Ophthalmol Otolaryngol, 76:*1444, 1972.

Quick, C.A.: Chemical and drug effects on inner ear. In Paparella, M.M., and Shumrick, D.A. (Eds.): *Otolaryngology.* Philadelphia, Saunders, 1973.

Ranck, J.B., Jr., and Windle, W.F.: Brain damage in the monkey, *Macaca mulata,* by asphyxia neonatorum. *Exp. Neurol, 1:*130, 1959.

Rasmussen, A.T.: Studies of the eighth cranial nerve of man. *Laryngoscope, 50:*67, 1940.

Rasmussen, G.L.: The olivary peduncle and other fiber projections of the superior olivary complex. *J Comp Neurol, 84:*141, 1946.

Rasmussen, G.L.: Selective silver impregnation of synaptic endings. In Windle, W.F. (Ed.): *New Research Techniques of Neuroanatomy.* Springfield, Thomas, 1957.

Rasmussen, G.L.: Efferent fibers of the cochlear nerve and cochlear nucleus. In Rasmussen, G.L., and Windle, W.F. (Eds.): *Neural Mechanisms of the Auditory and Vestibular Systems.* Springfield, Thomas, 1960.

Rasmussen, G.L.: Anatomic relationships of the ascending and descending auditory systems. In Fields, W.S., and Alford, B.R. (Eds.): *Neurological Aspects of Auditory and Vestibular Disorders.* Springfield, Thomas, 1964.

Rasmussen, G.L.: Efferent connections of the cochlear nucleus. In Graham, A.B. (Ed.): *Sensorineural Hearing Processes and Disorders.* Boston, Little, 1967.

Rintleman, W.F., Oyer, H.J., Forbord, J.L. et al.: Acupuncture as a treatment for sensorineural hearing loss. *Arch Otolaryngol, 99:*300, 1974.

Rose, J.E., and Galambos, R.: Microelectrode studies on medial geniculate body of cat. Thalamic region activated by click stimuli. *J Neurophysiol, 15:*343, 1952.

Rose, J.E., Galambos, R., and Hughes, J.: Organization of frequency sensitive neurons in the cochlear nuclear complex of the cat. In Rasmussen, G.L., and Windle, W.F. (Eds.): *Neural Mechanisms of the Auditory and Vestibular Systems.* Springfield, Thomas, 1960.

Rose, J.E., Greenwood, D.D., Goldberg, J.M. et al.: Some discharge characteristics of single neurons in the inferior colliculus of the cat. Tonotopical organization, relation of spike-counts to tone intensity, and firing patterns of single elements. *J Neurophysiol, 26:*294, 1963.

Rose, J.E., and Woolsey, C.N.: Cortical connections and functional organization of the thalamic auditory system of the cat. In Harlow, H.F., Woolsey, C.N. (Eds.): *Biological and Biochemical Bases of Behavior.* Madison, U of Wis Pr, 1958.

Rosen, S., and Rosen, H.V.: High frequency studies in school children in nine countries. *Laryngoscope, 81:*1007, 1971.

Rosenbluth, J.: The fine structure of acoustic ganglia in the rat. *J Cell Biol, 12:*329, 1962.

Ross, M.D.: Fluorescence and electron microscopic observations of the general visceral, efferent innervation of the inner ear. *Acta Otolaryngol, Suppl 286,* 1971.

Ross, M.D., and Burkel, W.: Multipolar neurons in the spiral ganglion of the rat. *Acta Otolaryngol, 76:*381, 1973.

Ruedi, L.: Histopathology of sensorineural degeneration and other inner ear changes in otosclerosis. In Schuknecht, H.F. (Ed.): *Otosclerosis.* Boston, Little, 1962.

Ruedi, L., and Spoendlin, H.: Pathogenesis of sensorineural deafness in otosclerosis. *Ann Otol, 75:*525, 1966.

Rydell, R.E., and Pulec, J.L.: Arnold-Chiari malformation. Neuro-otologic symptoms. *Arch Otolaryngol, 94:*8, 1971.

Saito, H., and Daly, J.F.: Quantitative analysis of acid mucopolysaccharides in the normal and kanamycin intoxicated cochlea. *Acta Otolaryngol, 71:*22, 1971.

Sando, I.: The anatomical interrelationships of the cochlear nerve fibers. *Acta Otolaryngol, 59:*417, 1965.

Sando, I., Bergstrom, L., Wood, R.P., II *et al.:* Temporal bone findings in trisomy 18 syndrome. *Arch Otolaryngol, 91:*552, 1970.

Sando, I., Black, F.O., Randolph, G. *et al.:* Lymphosarcoma invading the temporal bone contents. *Laryngoscope, 79:*2140, 1969.

Saxen, A.: Inner ear in presbycusis. *Acta Otolaryngol, 41:*213, 1952.

Saxena, R.K., Tandon, P.N., Sinha, A. *et al.:* Auditory functions in raised intracranial pressure. *Acta Otolaryngol, 68:*402, 1969.

Schindler, R.A., Lundquist, P.-G., and Morrison, M.D.: Endolymphatic sac response to cryosurgery of the lateral ampulla. *Ann Otol, 83:*674, 1974.

Schuknecht, H.F.: Techniques for study of cochlear function and pathology in experimental animals. Development of the anatomical frequency scale for the cat. *Arch Otolaryngol, 58:*377, 1953.

Schuknecht, H.F.: Presbycusis. *Laryngoscope, 65:*402, 1955.

Schuknecht, H.F.: Neuroanatomical correlates of auditory sensitivity and pitch discrimination in the cat. In Rasmussen, G.L., and Windle, W.F. (Eds.): *Neural Mechanisms of the Auditory and Vestibular Systems.* Springfield, Thomas, 1960.

Schuknecht, H.F.: Further observations on the pathology of presbycusis. *Arch Otolaryngol, 80:*369, 1964.

Schuknecht, H.F.: Temporal bone removal at autopsy. Preparation and uses. *Arch Otolaryngol, 87:*129, 1968a.

Schuknecht, H.F.: Pathology of Meniere's disease. *Otolaryngol Clin N Am,* Oct, 1968b.

Schuknecht, H.F.: Mechanisms of inner ear injury from blows to the head. *Ann Otol, 78:*253, 1969.

Schuknecht, H.F.: *Pathology of the Ear.* Cambridge, Harvard Univ Pr, 1974.

Schuknecht, H.F., Allam, A.F., and Murakami, Y.: Pathology of secondary malignant tumors of the temporal bone. *Ann Otol, 77:*5, 1968.

Schuknecht, H.F., Benitez, J., Beekhuis, J. *et al.:* The pathology of sudden deafness. *Laryngoscope, 72:*1142, 1962.

Schuknecht, H.F., Churchill, J.A., and Doran, R.: The localization of acetylcholinesterase in the cochlea. *Arch Otolaryngol, 69:*549, 1959.

Schuknecht, H.F., and El Seifi, T.: Experimental observations on fluid physiology of inner ear. *Ann Otol, 72:*687, 1963.

Schuknecht, H.F., Igarashi, M., and Gacek, R.R.: The pathological types of cochleo-saccular degeneration. *Acta Otolaryngol, 59:*154, 1965.

Schuknecht, H.F., Watanuki, K., Takahashi, T. *et al.:* Atrophy of the stria vascularis, a common cause for hearing loss. *Laryngoscope, 84:*1777, 1974.

Schuknecht, H.F., and Woellner, R.C.: An experimental and clinical study of deafness from lesions of the cochlear nerve. *J Laryngol, 69:*75, 1955.

Schulz, R.A., and Hilding, D.A.: Nerve fiber growth and myelination in von Recklinghausen eighth nerve tumor. *J Neuropathol Exp Neurol, 29:*105, 1970.

Shambaugh, G.E., Jr.: *Surgery of the Ear,* Ed. II. Philadelphia, Saunders, 1967a.

Shambaugh, G.E., Jr.: Another syndrome of familial hereditary deafness. *Arch Otolaryngol, 86:*1, 1967b.

Shambaugh, G.E., Jr.: Observations on the endolymphatic sac in cases of hydrops. *Arch Otolaryngol, 89:*98, 1969.

Shambaugh, G.E., Jr. (Moderator of panel discussion): Diagnosis and treatment of cochlear otosclerosis. *Arch Otolaryngol, 97:*30, 1973.

Silverstein, H.: The inner ear fluids in man. *Laryngoscope, 83:*79, 1973.

Silverstein, H., Naufal, P., and Belal, A.: Causes of elevated perilymph protein concentration. *Laryngoscope, 83:*476, 1973.

Simmons, F.B.: Cochlear microphonics and endolymph fistulas. *Otolaryngol Clin N Am,* Oct, 1968.

Simmons, F.B., Mongeon, C.J., Lewis, W.R. *et al.:* Electrical stimulation of acoustical nerve and inferior colliculus. Results in man. *Arch Otolaryngol, 79:*559, 1964.

Skinner, H.A.: Origin of acoustic nerve tumors. *Br J Surg, 16:*440, 1929.

Smith, C.A.: Vascular patterns of the membranous labyrinth. In de Lorenzo, A.J.D. (Ed.): *Vascular Disorders and Hearing Defects.* Baltimore, Univ Park Pr, 1973.

Smith, C.A., and Haglan, B.J.: Golgi stains on the guinea pig organ of Corti. *Acta Otolaryngol, 75:*203, 1973.

Smith, C.A., Lowry, O.H., and Wu, M.-L.: The electrolytes of the labyrinthine fluids. *Laryngoscope, 64:*141, 1954.

Snow, J.B., Jr.: Sudden deafness. In Paparella, M.M., and Shumrick, D.A. (Eds.): *Otolaryngology.* Philadelphia, Saunders, 1973.

Snow, J.B., Jr., and Suga, F.: Control of cochlear blood flow. In de Lorenzo, A.J.D. (Ed.): *Vascular Disorders and Hearing Defects.* Baltimore, Univ Park Pr, 1973.

Spector, G.J., and Carr, C.: The electron transport system in the cochlear hair cell: The ultrastructural cytochemistry of respiratory enzymes in hair cell mitochondria of the guinea pig. *Laryngoscope, 84:*1673, 1974.

Spector, G.J., and Lucente, F.E.: Aerobic metabolism of the inner ear: results of a critical evaluation. *Laryngoscope, 84:*1663, 1974.

Spencer, J.T., Jr.: Hyperlipoproteinemias in the etiology of inner ear disease. *Laryngoscope, 83:*639, 1973.

Spoendlin, H.: The innervation of the organ of Corti. *J Laryngol, 87:*717, 1967.

Spoendlin, H.: Ultrastructure and peripheral innervation pattern of the receptor in relation to the first coding of the acoustic message. In De Reuck, A.V.S., and Knight, J. (Eds.): *Hearing Mechanisms in Vertebrates.* Boston, Little, 1968.

Spoendlin, H.: Innervation patterns in the organ of Corti of the cat. *Acta Otolaryngol, 67:*239, 1969.

Spoendlin, H.: Degeneration behavior of the cochlear nerve. (In English)

*Arch klin exp Ohr-, Nas-u Kehlk Heilk, 200:*275, 1971.

Spoendlin, H.: Innervation densities of the cochlea. *Acta Otolaryngol, 73:* 235, 1972.

Spoendlin, H.: Autonomic nerve supply to the inner ear. In de Lorenzo, A.J.D. (Ed.): *Vascular Disorders and Hearing Defects.* Baltimore, Univ Park Pr, 1973.

Spoendlin, H., and Brun, J.P.: Relation of structural damage to exposure time and intensity in acoustic trauma. *Acta Otolaryngol, 75:*220, 1973.

Spoendlin, H., and Gacek, R.R.: Electronmicroscopic study of the efferent and afferent innervation of the organ of Corti in the cat. *Ann Otol, 72:* 660, 1963.

Stack, C.R., and Webster, D.B.: Glycogen content in the outer hair cells of kangaroo rat (*D. spectabilis*) cochlea prior to and following auditory stimulation. *Acta Otolaryngol, 71:*483, 1971.

Stotler, W.A.: An experimental study of the cells and connections of the superior olivary complex of the cat. *J Comp Neurol, 98:*401, 1953.

Strauss, M., and Davis, G.L.: Viral disease of the labyrinth. Review of the literature and discussion of the role of cytomegalovirus in congenital deafness. *Ann Otol, 82:*577, 1973.

Strominger, N.L.: Projections of the dorsal cochlear nucleus in the Rhesus monkey. (Abstract) *Anat Rec, 163:*271, 1969.

Strominger, N.L., and Oesterreich, R.E.: Localization of sound after section of the brachium of the inferior colliculus. *J Comp Neurol, 138:*1, 1970.

Strominger, N.L., and Strominger, A.I.: Ascending brain stem projections of the anteroventral cochlear nucleus in the Rhesus monkey. *J Comp Neurol, 143:*217, 1971.

Suga, F., Nakashima, T., and Snow, J.B.: Sodium and potassium ions in endolymph. *In vivo* measurements with glass electrodes. *Arch Otolaryngol, 91:*37, 1970.

Suga, F., Preston, J., and Snow, J.B., Jr.: Experimental microembolization of cochlear vessels. *Arch Otolaryngol, 92:*213, 1970.

Sugar, J.O., Engström, H., and Stahle, J.: Stria vascularis. *Acta Otolaryngol, Suppl, 301,* 1972.

Sugiura, S., and Paparella, M.M.: The pathology of labyrinthine ossification. *Laryngoscope, 77:*1974, 1967.

Suh, K.W., and Cody, D.T.: Obliteration of vestibular and cochlear aqueducts in the guinea pig. *Laryngoscope, 84:*1352, 1974.

Tarlov, I.M.: Structure of the nerve root. Nature of the junction between the central and peripheral nervous system. *Arch Neurol Psychiatry, 37:* 555, 1937.

Taylor, R.W.: Nonchromaffin paraganglioma, tympanic and jugulare. *Arch Otolaryngol, 68:*562, 1958.

Terplan, K.L., Sandberg, A.A., and Aceto, T., Jr.: Structural anomalies in the cerebellum in association with trisomy. *J A M A, 197:*557, 1966.

Thalman, R., Miyoshi, T., and Thalmann, I.: The influence of ischemia upon the energy reserves of inner ear tissues. *Laryngoscope, 82:*2249, 1972.

Thalmann, R., Thalmann, I., and Comegys, T.H.: Quantitative cytochemistry of the organ of Corti: Dissection, weight determination and analysis of single outer hair cells. *Laryngoscope, 82:*2059, 1972.

Truex, R.C., and Carpenter, M.B.: *Human Neuroanatomy,* Ed. VI. Baltimore, Williams & Wilkins, 1969.

van Noort, J.: The anatomical basis for frequency analysis in the cochlear nuclear complex. (In English) *Psychiatr Neurol Neurochir, 72:*109, 1969.

Ward, P.H.: The histopathology of auditory and vestibular disorders in head traumas. *Ann Otol, 78:*227, 1969.

Ward, P.H., Honrubia, V., and Moore, B.S.: Inner ear pathology in deafness due to maternal rubella. *Arch Otolaryngol, 87:*22, 1968.

Ward, W.D.: Noise-induced hearing damage. In Paparella, M.M., and Shumrick, D.A. (Eds.): *Otolaryngology.* Philadelphia, Saunders, 1973.

Ward, W.D., and Duvall, A.J., III: Behavioral and ultrastructural correlates of acoustic trauma. *Ann Otol, 80:*881, 1971.

Webster, D.B.: Projection of the cochlea to cochlear nuclei in Merriam's kangaroo rat. *J Comp Neurol, 143:*323, 1971.

Wever, E.G., Lawrence, M., Hemphill, R.W. *et al.:* The effects of oxygen deprivation upon the cochlear potentials. *Am J Physiol, 159:*199, 1949.

Whitfield, I.C.: *The Auditory Pathway.* London, Edward Arnold, 1967.

Williams, H.L.: Definition of terms in Meniere's disease. *Otolaryngol Clin N Am,* Oct, 1968.

Williamson, D.G., and Gifford, D.F.: Psychomatic aspects of Meniere's disease. *Acta Otolaryngol, 72:*118, 1971.

Wilson, S.A.K.: In Bruce, A.N. (Ed.): *Neurology.* Baltimore, Williams & Wilkins, 1940.

Winther, F.O.: X-ray irradiation of the inner ear of the guinea pig. An electron microscopic study of the degenerating outer hair cells of the organ of Corti. *Acta Otolaryngol, 69:*61, 1970.

Wolf, A., and Cowen, D.: Perinatal infections of the central nervous system. In Minckler, J. (Ed.): *Pathology of the Nervous System.* New York, McGraw, 1972.

Wolff, D., Bernhard, W.G., Tsutsumi, S. *et al.:* The pathology of Cogan's syndrome causing profound deafness. *Trans Am Otol Soc, 53:*94, 1965.

Woolsey, C.N., and Walzl, E.M.: Topical projection of nerve fibers from local regions of the cochlea to the cerebral cortex of the cat. *Johns Hopkins Hosp Bull, 71:*315, 1942.

INDEX

Hurler's syndrome, 121
Hydrops, endolymphatic, 39, 133, 202
Hyperostosis, foramina of osseous lamina
  cribrosa, 201
Hypertension, 183
Hypoglycemia, 40

I

Infections with molds, 129
  parasitic, 133
Inferior colliculus, 16, 75, 93
Influenza, 132
Inhibition, auditory, 94
Injury, head, 143
Internal auditory meatus, 18, 21, 50, 161
Intoxication, medicinal, 154
Intracranial pressure, increased, 157
Intraganglionic spiral bundle, 48, 94
Irradiation, laser, 153
  penetrating, 153

K

Kernicterus, 108
Klippel-Feil syndrome, 121

L

Labyrinth, 18
  membranous, 11, 23
  osseous, 19
Labyrinthine artery, 52
  bone, 15, 22
  fluids, 37
  ossification, 22, 103, 196
  osteoporosis, 196
Labyrinthitis, 123
  purulent, 127
  serous, 123
  viral, 129
Laceration, 144
Lamina cribrosa, 21, 52
  spiral, 23, 45
    osseous, 21
Laser irradiation, 153
Lateral lemniscus, 92
Leukemia, 169
Ligament, spiral—*see* Spiral crest
Limbus, spiral, 32, 37
Lipid metabolism, 197
Loudness recruitment, 47, 100, 113

Lupus-polyarteritis-rheumatic disorders,
  135
Lymphoma, 169

M

Maldevelopment, types, 105
Measles, 131
Meatus, internal auditory, 18, 21, 50
Medial geniculate body, 16, 82, 93
Medicinal intoxication, 154
Melanocytes, 50
Membrane, basilar, 14, 21, 23, 25, 34, 45
  Reissner's—*see* Vestibular membrane
  reticular, 34
  round window, 23
  tectorial, 34, 37
  vestibular, 11, 22, 25, 38
Membranous labyrinth, 11, 23
Meniere's syndrome, 133, 141, 201
Meningioma, 165
Meningitis, 127
Metastatic tumors, 172
Modiolus, 15, 21, 40
Mumps, 129
Myeloma, 169

N

Nerve, acoustic, 50
  cochlear, 21, 50, 58
    tonotopic structure, 51
Nerves, efferent, 47
Nerve fibers, adrenergic, 50
  cochlear, 40
  structures, efferent, acetylcholinester-
    ase in, 48
  supply to hair cells, 42
    organ of Corti, 42, 45, 48
Nerve, vestibular, 50
Neuritis, toxic, 125
Neurofibroma, 160
Neuronitis, vestibular, 205
Neurons, cochlear, 40
Norepinephrine, 29
  in glomus jugulare tumor, 172
Nuclear complex, dorsal olivary, 69
Nuclei of lateral lemniscus, 69, 73
Nucleus, cochlear, 16, 50, 55
  cell types, 61

Stimulus, acoustic, 34
Striae, auditory, 90
Stria vascularis, 27, 38, 39
   atrophy in presbycusis, 177
Sulcus, spiral, 29, 32
Supporting cells, 42
Synaptic terminals in cochlear nucleus, 58
Syphilis, 133

T

Tectorial membrane, 34, 37
Teratoma, 169
Thalamus, 17
Thalidomide, ingestion, 113
Thyroid dysfunction, 195
Tonotopic frequency structure, cochlea, 96
   cochlear nerve, 51
      nucleus, 96
   cortex, auditory, 98
   inferior colliculus, 98
   medial dorsal olivary nucleus, 97
      geniculate body, 98
Toxic encephalitis, 125
   neuritis, 125
Toxoplasmosis, 108, 133
Tract projections and connections, 90
Tractus spirals foraminosus, 50
Transsynaptic cell degeneration, 101
Trapezoid body, 90
   nucleus, 69, 73
Trauma, acoustic, 145

Tumor, glomus jugulare, 169
Tumors, cerebellopontine recess, 159
   metastatic, 172
Tunnel, outer, 32

U

Ultrasound, 151
Usher's syndrome, 120
Utricle, 11, 19
Utricular duct, 11, 22

V

Variation in normal cell population, 101
Venous return, labyrinth, 53
Vertigo of central origin, 205
Vestibule, 19, 22
Vestibular aqueduct, 15, 18, 19, 22, 39
   membrane, 11, 22, 25, 38
   nerve, 50
   neuronitis, 205
Viral disease, cytomegalic, 108
   labyrinthitis, 129
Vulnerability, zonal, cochlea and cochlear nucleus, 99

W

Window, oval, 19
   round, 19, 22

Z

Zonal vulnerability, cochlea and cochlear nucleus, 99